PERSPECTIVES

A GP reflects on medical practice
and, well, just about everything . . .

Judith Harvey started her career as a research scientist. Then, after running VSO's Papua New Guinea programme and teaching in a comprehensive school in Liverpool, she applied to medical school. She has been a partner, a locum and a salaried GP, and was a medical politician, chairing her Local Medical Committee and sitting on the General Practitioners Committee of the BMA. In 2010 she founded Cuba Medical Link, a registered charity which enabled around 400 medical students to go to Cuba for their electives.

As an SHO in Obs and Gynae she co-authored a book entitled *Cervical Cancer and How to Stop Worrying about It.* Since then she has written extensively about sessional GPs and patient involvement in books and GP journals, and for 10 years has contributed a blog for the newsletter of the National Association of Sessional GPs. This book is a collection of those and other articles.

PERSPECTIVES

A GP reflects on medical practice
and, well, just about everything . . .

Judith Harvey

Random Thoughts Limited
London

Harvey, Judith
Perspectives

British Library Cataloguing-in-Publication Data

A catalogue record for this book is available from the British Library

ISBN 978-0-9513573-8-5

Published in Great Britain 2018

Published by
  Random Thoughts Limited
  1 Bell Street, 2nd Floor
  London, NW1 5BY
  Email: info@randomthoughtslimited.co.uk
  Website: www.randomthoughtslimited.co.uk

This book has been designed by Jon Anderson, www.idstream.eu

Cover photograph: The author on the South West Coast Path
© Chuck Anderson

Foreword

In 2006 Dr Richard Fieldhouse, the founder and chairman of the National Association of Sessional GPs, asked me to review a book for the Association's newsletter. For the next edition I offered Richard an article about one-time medical student Hector Berlioz. Since then I have filled the back page of every issue, writing on anything from wart-charming to robots.

So, this book is a collection of ten years of meditations on health and medical matters in the widest sense. These 74 short articles were written for an audience of GPs but hopefully will be of interest to anyone, professional or patient – and we are all sometimes patients.

Where colleagues and actual patients other than myself are referred to, identifying features have been changed to protect their privacy.

Judith Harvey

Acronyms

ADHD	Attention Deficit Hyperactivity Disorder
BMA	British Medical Association (doctors' professional association and trade union)
BMJ	British Medical Journal
BNF	British National Formulary (information about all medications)
CJD	Creutzfeldt-Jakob Disease
DRCOG	Diploma of the Royal College of Obstetrics and Gynaecology
ECG	Electrocardiogram (heart tracing)
ECT	Electroconvulsive therapy (still used for severe depression)
ENT	Ear Nose and Throat (surgical specialty)
FRCS	Fellow of the Royal College of Surgeons
GMC	General Medical Council (licenses doctors to practice and sets standards for education and professional conduct)
GPC	General Practitioners Committee of the BMA (represents all GPs in policy making and negotiating with the government)
ITU/ICU	Intensive Therapy/Care Unit
LMC	Local Medical Committee (elected body of GPs which represents all GPs in an area)
?MI	Does this patient have a Myocardial Infarct? (heart attack) – a common entry in medical records
MRCP	Member of the Royal College of Physicians
MRSA	Methicillin-resistant Staphylococcus aureus (a bacterial superbug)
MSF	Médecins Sans Frontières
NASGP	National Association of Sessional GPs (campaigning and support organisation of GPs who work as locums or who are employed rather than being partners in a practice)
NGO	Non-governmental Organisation
O/E NAD	On Examination Nothing Abnormal Discovered
PSA	Prostatic Specific Antigen (blood test used for screening and monitoring prostate cancer)
PTSD	Post-traumatic Stress Disorder
QOF codes	Quality and Outcomes Framework (tick-box system introduced in 2004 aiming to improve the quality of care, now abolished in Scotland)
RCGP	Royal College of GPs
RTA	Road Traffic Accident
SHO	Senior House Officer
SLE	Systemic Lupus Erythematosus (an autoimmune disease)
UTI	Urinary Tract Infection (most commonly cystitis)
VSO	Voluntary Service Overseas
VTS	Vocational Training Scheme (for GPs)
WHO	World Health Organisation

To Richard Fieldhouse,
who gave me the opportunity,
and to my husband, Chuck Anderson,
who gave me the support.

Contents

VII Careers

VIII Politics

IX Future

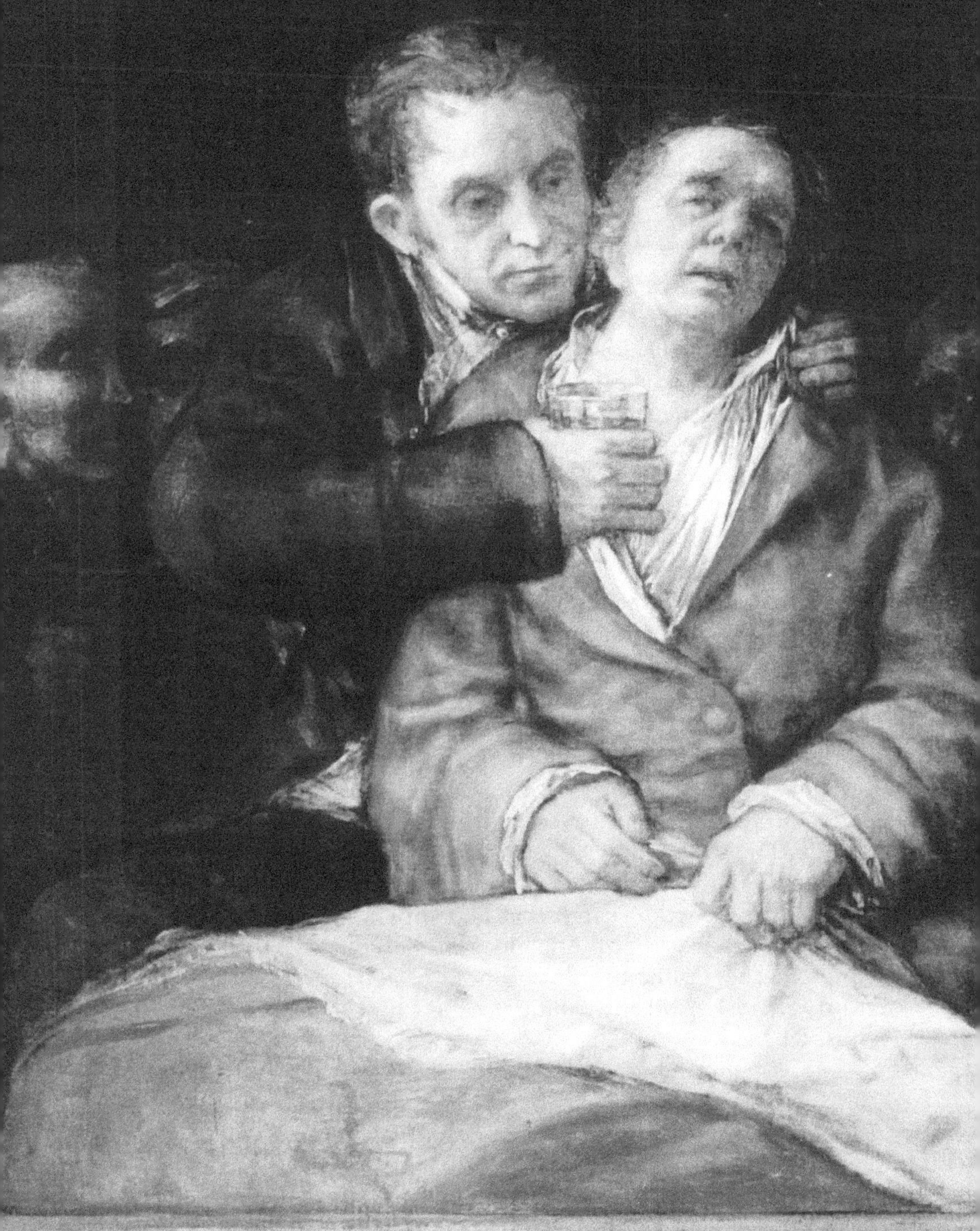

oya agradecido, á su amigo Arrieta: por el acierto y esmero con q.e le salvó la vida en su agu
eligrosa enfermedad, padecida á fines del año 1819 a los setenta y tres de su edad. Lo pintó en

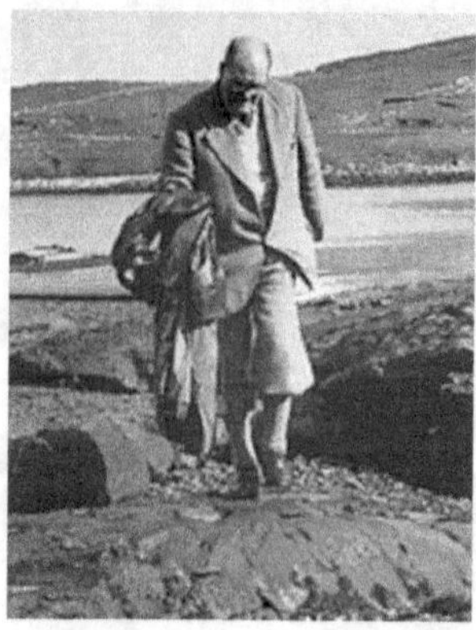

An Dotair Mòr

GP sought to establish first practice on island. No electricity. No telephone. Nearest hospital 12 hours away by boat, weather permitting. Obstetric skills and Gaelic essential.

That, in essence, was what The Highlands and Islands Medical Service was offering. Plus a house, a rowing boat and a car (of limited use as there were few roads), and a basic income so that the doctor could afford to treat those who couldn't give even a chicken in payment.

Dr Alexander Macleod took up the post in the Outer Hebrides in 1932. He was responsible for 3,000 people on North Uist and 16 outer islands, some home to as few as two families. He'd spent a year in Antarctica, then worked as a locum in cities and rural areas. As we know, this teaches you flexibility and independence. But he didn't find his new job easy. He later admitted that at first moving to North Uist felt like a big mistake. He was always finding fault. Then he realised that it was he that was out of tune with island life, and he settled down.

Islanders' health was very poor. Isolated from the rest of the world, they relied on each other and superstition. TB and measles were rife. So was diphtheria: one family had lost four children in three weeks. Public health was non-existent. So there was much to do. And he did it. A patient called him 'a one-man walking hospital'.

An Dotair Mòr – the big doctor, as he was known – was always available. He was a witness to his patients' lives and their sufferings. He understood that medical and social needs are inseparable. He knew when to look for the real reason for a consultation; patients' body language, he said, was "straws which show which way the wind is blowing".

He never refused a visit. Emergency requests were delivered by a messenger or in Morse code via the single wire which ringed North Uist. He would travel by car, boat, horse, tractor, and on foot. A lantern or a white sheet would signal that a tractor should come and pick him up. Once he had to swim for it when the boat foundered.

In 1932, patients who needed urgent hospital care faced a long, uncomfortable journey by sea to Glasgow. Dr Alex persuaded the *Daily Record* to sponsor a mercy flight and in 1933 a biplane first landed on the beach. The air ambulance service is one of his many legacies. It didn't just take ill patients to hospital; it brought back the dying to spend their last days at home.

He delivered 2,000 babies, including John Gillies, future chair of the Scottish RCGP, and the techniques he devised for managing obstetric emergencies unaided were published in the BMJ and widely adopted. When childhood immunisation was introduced in 1955 he tested it on his own children before persuading the islanders to accept it.

He served North Uist for 40 years. His wife, Dr Julia, was also a GP. She ran the practice, milked the cows and stood in when her husband was out visiting a patient or away challenging authority at meetings. One January night in 1935 she went to help a nurse with a difficult delivery. The visit involved a 45-minute boat trip and a two-mile walk there and then back again after the successful delivery. Two days later she herself gave birth to the first of their five children.

When Dr Alex retired, aged 80, his son Dr John and daughter-in-law Lorna, a nurse, carried on the tradition of service to the community. Dr John held educational meetings with local fisherman and emergency services, and secured legislation for sailors to wear life jackets when he realised that several fishermen had fallen overboard and drowned when they took a pee over the side. Like his father, he fostered contact with the wider world and in 1998 hosted a meeting of the World Organisation of Family Doctors on the tiny island of Berneray.

Were the Macleods the doctors of the past or of the future? Dr Alex was independent in a way that is impossible today. He could be autocratic, but he had to think for himself. He challenged accepted dogma, but he didn't much like being challenged himself, though he worked closely with the district nurses, and a nurse who questioned him found a box of chocolates handed round the door next morning. He could be imperious. Driving around the island's single-track roads he would never pull into a passing place; that was for others to do. Crusty and gruff he could be, but he knew the meaning of service and he was beloved by his patients, respected by all, and a role model for the medical students and young doctors he encouraged to spend time in his practice. His memory is still very much alive on Uist and he must be a hard act for his 21st-century successors to follow.

These days you are never far from a *caffè latte* in the Outer Hebrides, and the mobile cinema brings blockbusters to isolated communities. As long as the power supply is working. But the islands still find it hard to recruit and keep GPs. The winters are long, the wind blows year around and the population has halved since 1932 .

Even in summer the Outer Hebrides feel like another country. In North Uist in August the post-bus picked us up at the end of a walk. The postman hadn't finished his deliveries, and he warned us that the 15-mile journey might take a couple of hours. We stopped to deliver a letter addressed to 'The Nurse's House'. It was where the nurse had lived in Dr Alex's time. We drove down rough lanes to outlying crofts. The postman parked the van on the grass and riffled through the box of mail at our feet – bills, Amazon deliveries, *Private Eye*. Householders emerged for a chat, usually in Gaelic, before we drove on to the next croft. On the winding coastline near Clachan, facing the Atlantic Ocean, we came to a striking stone memorial. Erected by their patients, it commemorates the Macleods with the inscription '*Choimhlion iad an dleasdanas gu buileach*' – 'They excelled in their duties'.

—NASGP December 2015

Photo: © Neil Preismann

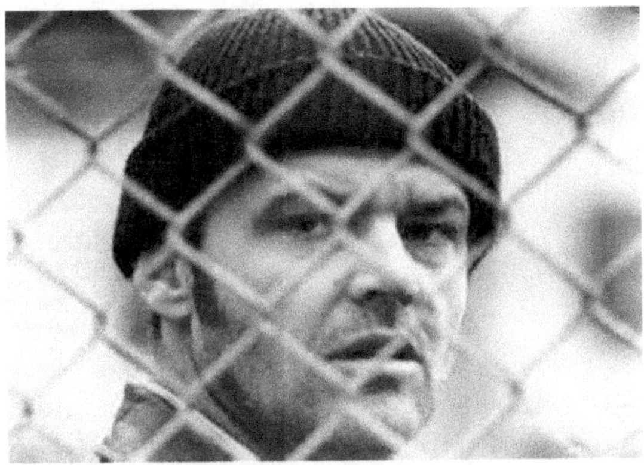

The Cuckoo's Nest

The BMJ doesn't often publish obituaries of provincial American doctors. But it gave Dean Brooks a full-page send-off. Why?

From 1955 till 1981 Dean Brooks was superintendent of Oregon State Hospital. That's where they filmed *One Flew Over the Cuckoo's Nest*. It's a 1975 classic film. It tells the story of Randle McMurphy, a petty criminal who decides it might be more comfortable to serve out his sentence for statutory rape in a hospital rather than doing hard labour in prison. He, and we, find out how wrong he was, and he ends up, well, I won't spoil the story but in his defeat he has enabled someone else to live. The film won five Oscars and made Jack Nicholson a superstar.

Back to Dean Brooks. The book from which the film was (quite faithfully) taken was published in 1962 and set in Oregon State Hospital. Ten years later Hollywood producers called to say they would like to make the film there. Brooks was interested. He felt strongly about the dignity of psychiatric patients and saw it as a chance to advocate for the mentally ill. And he thought it would be fun. He discussed the proposal with patients. They were keen. His fellow doctors were ambivalent. The hospital authorities were adamant: they forbade him to speak to the film people. So he didn't. But his wife did. As Brooks said, "It's easier to ask for forgiveness than permission".

Brooks insisted that the patients be treated with respect, and that members of the film team, including the director and scriptwriter, spend time with the patients. The crew lived in the hospital before filming started, and during the 14 weeks of filming the actors lived there too. They stayed in role during breaks from filming. When Jack Nicholson arrived, he couldn't tell them from the patients.

Around 90 patients took part in the filming. The director asked Brooks to read for the part for hospital superintendent. Brooks threw down the stilted script, and he and Jack Nicholson ad-libbed their scenes together. They are brilliant. Also unscripted was a scene where McMurphy's future care is discussed by the doctors, mostly played by psychiatrists at the hospital, and the chief nurse, the chilling Nurse Ratched. Louise Fletcher's performance won her an Oscar.

In the 1960s patients admitted with acute mental problems were housed together with long-stay patients with developmental problems. The film could have been a freak show. But it isn't, although most doctors will recognise patients from their days in psychiatric units. They will recognise the group therapy sessions. They will recognise the doctors' and nurse's discussion of McMurphy's mental state.

For the anti-psychiatry movement, the film was a gift. The group sessions, led with deceptive reasonableness by Nurse Ratched, may initially appear therapeutic. But as they develop, and particularly when McMurphy challenges her authority, they are instruments of coercion and control. If that doesn't cow the patient, the next punishment for insubordination to her regime is ECT without anaesthesia. The ultimate threat for those who fail to conform to rigid ward rules is lobotomy, and the patients know it.

Brooks was aware that *Cuckoo's Nest* could be used as a weapon against psychiatry. He insisted that the film be set in 1962, when the book was published, with a disclaimer pointing out that by 1975 psychiatry had moved on from the regimes depicted in the film. Brooks saw that the story is an allegory about power and how it is abused in any institution.

The film's message is as relevant as ever. How many hospital superintendents in 2013 would welcome a film crew making a feature film like *Cuckoo's Nest* into their hospital? I can't see any chief executives allowing it. And any doctor making the case for filming would quickly be subject to gagging, the modern contractual version of ECT. True, psychiatric care has changed. Nevertheless, chemical coshes are still used to control patients for the convenience of society.

Are there any institutions which don't seek to smother dissent? The talk in the prison service may be about rehabilitation but the reality is about control. And how many care homes manage to put the dignity of frail elderly residents above institutional needs? As in everyday life, it is very hard to counter passive aggression, and the easiest strategy is to submit.

In an interview recorded a few months before he died, Dean Brooks describes what putting patients first meant for him. When he went to Oregon in 1955, most psychiatric patients were obliged to wear identical baggy outfits. Brooks' patients wore their own clothes. They were sleeping in lighted dormitories. Brooks ordered that the lights be turned off at night so they could sleep better. Every opportunity was taken to break down barriers between the hospital and the community. He set up a task force of ten patients, ten staff and ten members of the community. He organised a 16-day wilderness hike for 51 chronic patients and 51 members of staff, an exercise in shared survival which proved transforming for relationships between patients and staff and healing for a substantial number of the participants.

Up to his death he campaigned for the decriminalisation of mental illness. And, something that particularly struck me, he always sorted his mail into piles, then opened letters from patients first. He left mail from managers to the last.

A remarkable man, remarkably memorialised in an Oscar-winning Hollywood film.

—NASGP October 2013

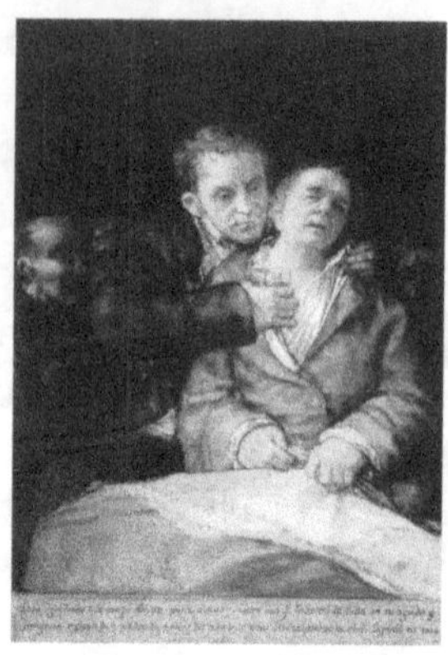

Portrait of a Doctor

Doctors don't feature much in art. True, the walls of Royal Colleges record changing fashions in portraiture, and wealthy society doctors like to commission pictures of themselves. Satirists like Hogarth have lampooned the quacks and moody Scandinavians included them as bit players in deathbed scenes. But only rarely does a picture featuring a doctor command our attention.

In his seventies, deaf and widowed, Francisco Goya was living at *Quinta del Sordo* (the Deaf Man's Farmhouse) near Madrid and covering its walls with his nightmare visions. Now known as the black paintings, they hang today in the Prado in Madrid. He fell ill and was attended by his friend Dr Eugenio García Arrieta. He recovered, and the next year painted *Goya curado por el doctor Arrieta* (*Goya Cured by Doctor Arrieta*) as a thank-you for his friend.

Goya's self-portrait shows how ill he was. His skin is grey, his eyes sunken, his jaw slack. He plucks at the sheets. Behind the two men other faces are faintly visible; perhaps Goya is hallucinating. He has no strength. Arrieta, his arm round the painter, props him up and urges him to drink. The liquid in the glass is brownish. Is it medicine, or perhaps wine which may well have been a safer fluid to take than water? The doctor's expression is intense; he has his eyes on the glass as he lifts it to Goya's lips. At this moment he is not permitting himself to yield to sorrow.

Arrieta was not the sort of quack that Goya himself mercilessly satirised in his aquatints *Los Caprichos*. He had apparently made a study of plague, and if so we can perhaps assume that he was a physician who made the best of his medical knowledge. In his dedication at the bottom of the painting Goya says his illness was 'acute and dangerous' and both men must have known that the painter, already 73, would in all probability succumb. In the inscription Goya acknowledges that his friend's skill and care saved his life.

Some see in Arrieta's face the benevolence of friendship, but I think that his expression conveys his anxiety for his patient's life, his fear that he cannot save him. The patient must take some fluids and he is intent on getting him to drink. But the doctor's anxiety is also that of a man whose friend is close to death. I think his compassion is shown not in his face but in his posture. He is physically and emotionally supporting the sick man. For the patient's sake he must tread the line between professionalism and friendship, and Goya's recovery is a testament to Arrieta's success in finding that delicate balance.

—NASGP August 2006

POSTSCRIPT (December 2015): I've just seen this picture again, in the National Gallery's exhibition of portraits by Goya. Goya was clearly too ill to be able to make a sketch at the time. So how did he produce such a realistic picture? Few artists can paint seriously ill people in a way that doctors recognise as lifelike. But Goya has succeeded – and in a self-portrait!

A READER WRITES: Dr Arrieta was born in 1770 in Cuéllar province of Segovia. In 1820 he was commissioned by the Spanish government to study 'the plague of the Levant' in the coast of Africa, where he probably died. Goya was 24 years older than his friend Arrieta, and the paradox is that he survived him eight years.

SEE ALSO: Photo reference to *Children of a Lesser God*, page 81.

Photo: *Self-portrait with Dr Arrieta,* also known as *Goya curado por el doctor Arrieta* was painted in 1820 by Francisco de Goya y Lucientes (1746-1828) and is in the Minneapolis Institute of the Arts

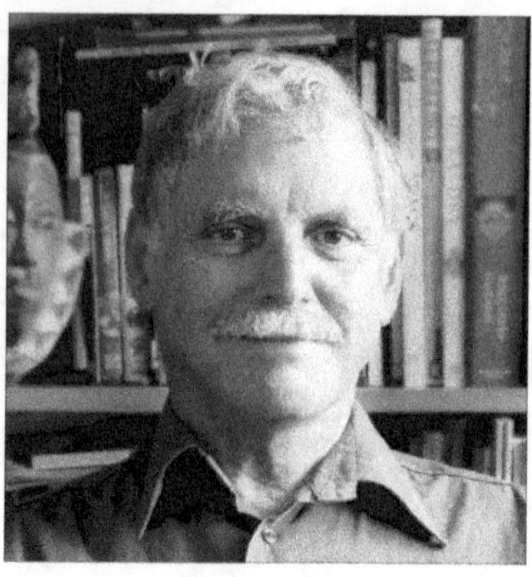

Suburban Shaman

The BMJ reviewer called it war poetry, Julia Neuberger wrote in *The Independent* that it should be required reading for every medical student, it's already been serialised on Radio 4. Cecil Helman's *Suburban Shaman* describes illness and its cultural context, and he writes from the front line – he was a GP for 27 years.

In the 1970s it was *A Fortunate Man*, a lyrical photojournalistic essay about the life and work – the two almost indistinguishable – of John Sassall, a rural GP, which shaped the aspirations of idealistic doctors. Is *Suburban Shaman* the *Fortunate Man* for a new generation – exploring the mystery of general practice in the London suburbs rather than in villages of the Forest of Dean?

Cecil Helman, scion of a medical family, came to London from his native South Africa in the late 1960s, primarily to escape serving in the army under the apartheid regime, but once here he escaped again – this time from his family history. He left medicine to study anthropology. When he returned to practice, he took his anthropological training with him, first on board a cruise liner as a ship's doctor, then into a consulting room in suburban London. Additionally, he has written a classic book, *Culture, Health and Illness*, and he runs a highly regarded course on cross-cultural primary care.

So *Suburban Shaman* has had a big build-up. Perhaps a degree of disappointment was inevitable. The first few chapters describe Helman's early life in South Africa. The anecdotes are interesting, but any liberal young South African exile of that era could produce a string of similar apartheid stories, and the immigrant's struggle with the contrast between Africa's big skies and 1960s London's cramped greyness has a familiar ring.

Helman went back to medicine and became a GP. His exposure in South Africa to other healing traditions, his anthropological training, and his own experience as a migrant and a patient illuminate his work. His stories are vivid, often amusing, sometimes sad.

His message is that patients seek a context for their illness, and this is what traditional systems of healing provide. Western medicine, with its goal of cure, has lost the art of healing, of relating the illness to the person and to their society. But if patients can understand why they are suffering they are better able to bear the uncertainty that even the most modern technical medicine cannot eliminate.

Helman acknowledges the place of hospitals and high-tech medicine, but he asks that we do not forget the person and their needs and hopes and fears and beliefs, and, like the shamans of his African childhood, that we bear witness to their travails.

If *Suburban Shaman* is the *Fortunate Man de nos jours*, what does that say about 2006? Certainly we live in less idealistic times than the 1960s. *Suburban Shaman* provides a humanistic conscience for an era in which intervention is expected to be evidence-based and subject to assessment by tick-box. Policy-makers pay heed!

A Fortunate Man today reads like an elegiac lament. It was written at a time when technological medicine was taking off and the social structures of generations were just beginning to crumble. Forty years on the 'suburban shaman' practises in a world which is irreversibly exiled from that imagined Eden. But there is still a place for inspirational role models. Maybe we act the suburban shaman during the week and dream on Sundays.

Nevertheless I would hold that the doctor-patient relationship, in general practice at least, is in no worse shape now than then. For every 'fortunate man' in 1967 there must have been many good-enough GPs struggling with work-life balance and a number of quacks ready to rip off the vulnerable.

In 2006 we may have abandoned 24-hour cover and will see few patients from cradle to grave, but our relationship with our patients is analysed by academics, examined in Balint groups, and dissected in VTS course sessions the length and breadth of the country. We recognise that the medium is at least as important as the message. Helman's message is thoughtful, and insightfully illustrated, but it isn't news.

And that is a good thing.

📖 ***Suburban Shaman: Tales from Medicine's Front Line***
Cecil Helman, 2006

📖 ***A Fortunate Man: The Story of a Country Doctor***
John Berger, 1967

—NASGP April 2006

Photo: Cecil Helman died in 2009

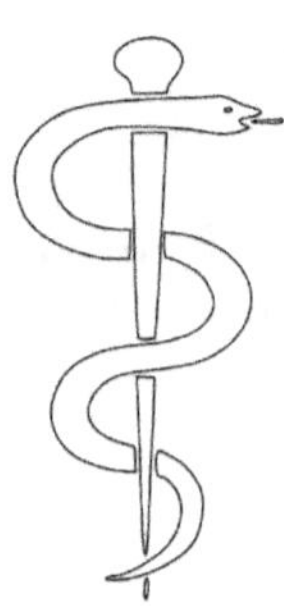

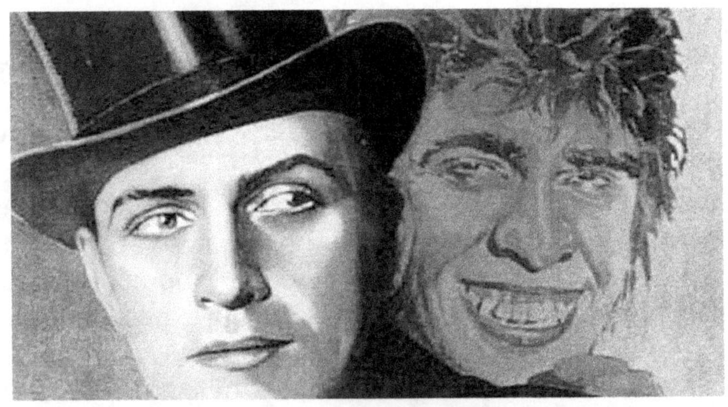

Dr Jekyll and Mr Hyde

A third-rate artist, a failed seminarian, a drop-out teacher. They don't sound a threatening trio. But between them they were responsible for the deaths of around 150 million people.

Neither Hitler, Stalin nor Mao were medical men. But some recent lesser tyrants were doctors: Haiti's Papa Doc Duvalier, Bosnian Serb Radovan Karadžić, and Bashar al-Assad of Syria among others.

Papa Doc's work on controlling yaws won him humanitarian accolades, but when he entered politics he was drawn into Haiti's voodoo culture and thousands lost their lives.

Radovan Karadžić was a psychiatrist with, apparently, a devoted following before he committed deeds for which he is now indicted for war crimes and genocide. His previous imprisonment for embezzlement suggests that his moral compass was adrift long before the Balkans sank into yet another ethnic conflict.

Reports on Bashar al-Assad's time at the Western Eye Hospital commend his kindly treatment of patients. His father's regime had lethally suppressed dissent, but Bashar appeared to have different values. Not now.

What turned these doctors? Belief that the cause for which they stood was worth the sacrifice of other peoples lives? French revolutionary Dr Jean-Paul Marat, who practised in Newcastle and St Andrews before joining the killing spree in Paris, thought so. Anyone who thinks Dr Che Guevara was an unblemished hero should investigate his involvement in the summary executions of prisoners during the Cuban revolutionary war and after it was won. The responsibilities and opportunities of power may have removed restraints which in normal times would have kept them on the straight and narrow.

Politicians can distance themselves from the unpleasant realities of killing other people, though some, like Papa Doc, discover a taste for sadism. Nazi doctors may not have seen themselves as sadistic: they viewed the people on whom they conducted their ghastly experiments as less than human. Doctors working on chemical and biological warfare in the Japanese army's Unit 731 may have felt the same about their victims. Should we make use of results obtained through such appalling experimentation? In the case of the Nazis, the ethical debate continues, but US general Douglas MacArthur had no such scruples: he granted the Japanese teams secret immunity in exchange for sharing their information with the Americans.

Are doctors as likely to be serial murderers in real life as they are in Agatha Christie's novels? Harold Shipman wasn't unique. In 1956 John Bodkin Adams was tried at the Old Bailey and acquitted of murdering two patients. He was reinstated by the GMC. Nevertheless, suspicion continued that he had killed around 160 old ladies, and was strengthened in 2003 when police archives were made public.

Other doctors have been charged with murdering a patient. Most believed they were acting to relieve suffering. Shipman is the only British doctor actually convicted of killing a patient. He didn't claim to be altruistic, and still no-one really knows what motivated him.

Doctors, like almost everyone else, can get sucked into the prevailing culture, whether it be that of African dictatorships or racist thugs. They can get swept up by ideologies. In their work they are always in a position of power: no amount of patient involvement can fully achieve an equal balance between the confident doctor and the vulnerable patient. Doctors have the means and the opportunity to administer harmful drugs. If the culture which keeps psychopathic tendencies buried is removed, a doctor may get high on the power of life and death. It's not surprising, either, that every now and again a doctor loses control and murders a family member.

What does this have to do with the rest of us? I think quite a lot. Doctors used to be put on pedestals, and they still retain public confidence. It's a deal: we demonstrate high professional and personal standards and in return we receive respect along with the bottle of Famous Grouse at Christmas. On a pedestal, you're exposed. Much is expected of you and you up your game.

But a doctor who is evil threatens this calculus. It sometimes feels like open season for doctor-bashing: the profession doesn't seem to be popular with the government, or with the *Daily Mail*. People in power would like to control doctors: downgrade them to technicians and gag them so they can't speak out. Stories about wicked doctors are a gift to them.

Can we identify the doctors who are going to turn bad? GPs Bodkin Adams and Shipman both had 'previous'; early in their careers both had been caught forging prescriptions for opiates. But it's easy to make firm diagnoses with a retrospectoscope.

Locums get an intimate view of other GPs' work. We work in their practices, we sit in their consulting rooms, we rummage in their desk drawers for equipment, we use their computers, we read their patients' records. What if we unearth empty gin bottles or murky websites, or notice odd prescribing habits or questionable clinical practice? Such GPs are most unlikely to be potential mass murderers, but they could be putting their patients at risk. All doctors have a duty to report colleagues if they feel their conduct gives cause for concern, and by shouldering our responsibilities we could help save a patient and even our profession.

—NASGP November 2013

SEE ALSO: *GP locums: When to Blow the Whistle?*, page 150

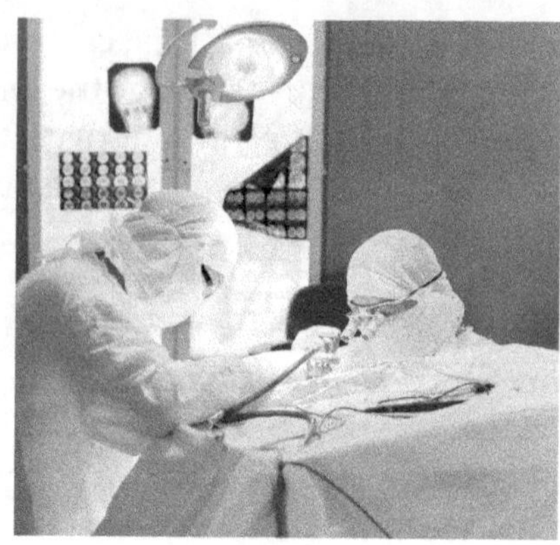

The Right Stuff?

There are doctors who work in war zones. There are doctors who spend their lives in laboratories. There are doctor-managers, doctor-novelists, doctor-comedians. A medical training can lead you almost anywhere. The trick is finding the niche which suits you.

The most high-octane branch of medicine in Britain is probably neurosurgery. The stakes are high and the risks, even of an apparently straightforward operation, are intimidating. Neurosurgeons can transform patients' lives, curing their brain tumour or rendering them a vegetable. Or both in the same operation. In general practice, every day there are things we could have done better, but we don't have to live with such catastrophic failures. How can anyone bear a lifetime on such a roller-coaster?

Henry Marsh knows. He's a neurosurgeon on the verge of retirement, and his memoir *Do no Harm* tells us what it's like.

Neurosurgeons need nerves of steel. If something goes wrong inside the patient's cranium you have to make split-second decisions. If you need time to make up your mind, take up dermatology.

We all live with guilt or shame about patients who suffered through our treatment, but it requires a particular resilience to walk through a care home recognising the names of patients who have been wrecked by your surgery, and then go back to the operating theatre.

As well as failure, doctors have to bear uncertainty. Even if the diagnosis is obvious – and that doesn't happen as often as medical soap operas suggest – the management of the problem is frequently less straightforward, despite all the protocols.

"Heal the sick, comfort the dying, and don't get them mixed up" doctor-novelist Colin Douglas was told many years ago by his consultant. Good advice, but the dividing line is often less clear now than it was then. And patients, and their families, may hold a different view of whether heroic treatment is still appropriate. Neurosurgeons may relish risk, but they have to navigate this quagmire as sensitively as do oncologists.

Every day clinicians walk a tightrope. Most of us stop noticing the drop, at least until we find ourselves up before the GMC. But some doctors leave clinical medicine because they cannot keep their balance over the abyss.

Patients still put doctors, particularly heroic surgeons, on a pedestal. But, like statues of Lenin, at any moment we may be pulled down and smashed. Henry Marsh has been criticised by readers for admitting to irritation in the supermarket queue. Maybe you need that touch of arrogance if you are to delve into someone else's brain. Better a bit of high-handedness if that hand has more skill and is willing to take on the difficult cases that a timid surgeon would turn down. GPs have less to be to arrogant about, but which of us hasn't felt frustrated when queuing to pay for our groceries, especially behind trolleys filled with junk food?

"You don't know what it's like" is a common criticism of doctors. It is another way of saying "You haven't shown me that you understand". Do doctors need to suffer what the patient is experiencing in order to understand? Henry Marsh's infant son had a brain tumour. It taught him what parents go through while he operates on their child. But personal experience doesn't guarantee empathy. It's easy to think "If I can put up with it, so can my patients".

Alternative practitioners don't have personal experience of every dis-ease, any more than doctors do, but they attract high approval ratings. Surely not because of their remedies. It's because their patients feel heard. What training do homeopaths have in consultation management, and why can't we doctors match them? Does the first year on the wards crush the learning from all those communication skills modules? Do we need more training in being nice? Or do we need more time to be nice?

Few alternative practitioners' consultation skills are tested by having to break terrible news. GPs break terrible news every so often, neurosurgeons every week. There is no right way to do it, just less bad ways, and however ruthless you are with a scalpel, to be a good doctor you must accomplish this most difficult of tasks with sensitivity and humility.

Of course patients want the perfect doctor. The GMC has compiled a daunting list of the virtues expected of us. But in the messy real world, everyone – government, patients, we ourselves – has to remember that perfection doesn't exist, and that what makes a doctor a good-enough brain surgeon is not what makes a good-enough GP.

There isn't one model for a good GP. The investment banker with sinusitis doesn't want his GP to probe his psyche, while for the downtrodden woman sinusitis is a ticket to a supportive listener. And we all have to learn. Someone has to be the first patient a trainee operates on or we wouldn't have doctors with the experience to tackle difficult cases.

The first thing doctors in clinical roles need is an interest in people. If you have that, doesn't all the rest follow? Add a smile and an analytical mind. So that you know when the patient needs tea and sympathy, and when it is time for coffee and a kick in the pants.

📖 ***Do No Harm: Stories of Life, Death and Brain Surgery***
Henry Marsh, 2014

—NASGP June 2014

SEE ALSO: *The Good, the Bad and the Ugly*, page 134

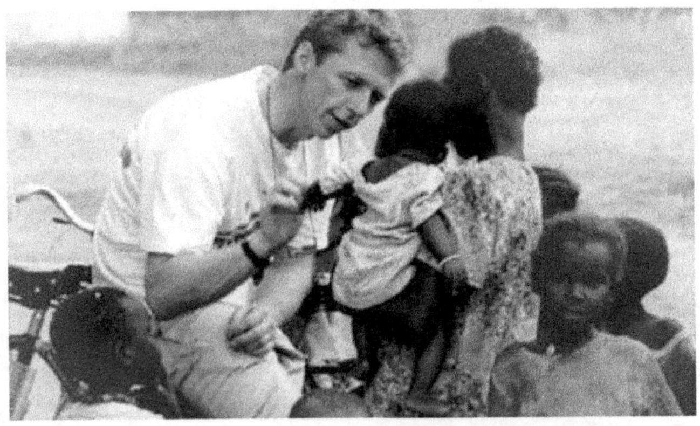

An Imperfect Offering

In 1999 James Orbinski went to Oslo to receive the Nobel Peace Prize on behalf of Médecins Sans Frontières. Born in Britain and brought up in Canada, it was at medical school that he found a focus for his nascent humanitarianism. And immunology captured his interest. Immunology led him to HIV, and HIV – this was the 1980s – led him to research in Africa. And Africa led him to Médecins Sans Frontières. To Somalia, Rwanda, Afghanistan, and eventually to Oslo. *An Imperfect Offering* is his account of those years.

Reading his book is like jolting along a terrible road in a nightmare. I struggled to keep everything straight in my head. So many places, so many people, so many acronyms. So much need. Who is doing what, and why? Who is on whose side? Can't he slow down and explain? No, he can't, because that's how it was. And one begins to experience the nightmare of hazardous journeys, living with the fear of what might be round the next corner. Living with the smell of faeces and vomit and recently butchered human beings. The smell of fear. The smell of horror: the woman systematically mutilated just enough so that she will bleed slowly to death, wild dogs tearing at human corpses, the little sausages scattered in the mud that turn out to be children's fingers.

Most books about inhumanity are leavened by examples of the human spirit transcending the horror. Very little in *An Imperfect Offering* enables one to close the book feeling good about being human. There seems to be no limit to man's ability to plan and execute cruelty – and to justify it.

When the Red Cross was founded in 1863 it was possible to

find a 'humanitarian space' between armies if one undertook, as the Red Cross did, to keep silent about the conflict. But a hundred years later silence seemed to kill more people than it saved. MSF was founded to speak out, but without taking sides. In the 21st century humanitarian assistance has become a political tool. Armies drop yellow parcels of cluster bombs on the 'bad' guys and a few miles away they drop yellow parcels of food on the 'good' guys. The children of both parties can't tell the difference between the parcels. Rich countries protect their interests – and improve their balance of payments – by selling arms to poor countries and ensuring that the international wheels run too slowly to stop the slaughter until their perceived ally has won. MSF can try to tell the world what is happening, although to continue giving humanitarian aid, it may have to pay protection money to warlords.

All a long way from the concerns of most of us here. But it is just as well to remember how so many people suffer, and that it is getting more difficult, not easier, to find the space in which they can be safely helped. And that the people who are courageous enough to go and help have to live with unremitting evidence of cruelty and with the decisions they made, not just in the field but for the rest of their lives.

In our safe world, too many people, too many managers, think that we should always be able to make the right decision. We step outside protocols and guidelines at our peril. But even in our 'safe' world it isn't like that. We may come to know after the event if we managed to take the less wrong decision, or we may never know. *An Imperfect Offering* is a salutary reminder that the world is an uncertain and a dangerous place. We may not all be called to speak out about a genocide, but calling the powerful to account is the duty of us all.

📖 ***An Imperfect Offering: Dispatches from the Medical Front Line*** *James Orbinski, 2008*

—NASGP October 2008

Photo: UCI Blum Center for Poverty Alleviation

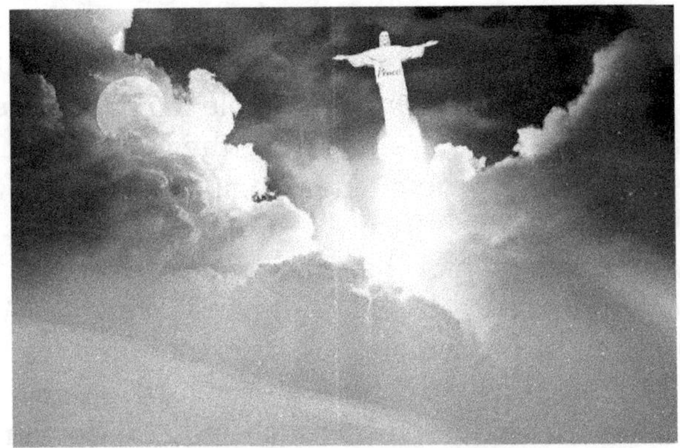

What Are the Rules in Hell?

Blood and Dust is a 30 minute video made in 2010 by former soldier and now independent video journalist (and sustainable farmer) Vaughan Smith about the work of a US Army air ambulance medivac team in Afghanistan.

Paramedics scramble out of a helicopter into a cloud of dust, clutching a stretcher. They re-emerge bearing a desperately injured marine. As the chopper swings into the air the paramedics have already started the life-saving protocol. In military medicine before ABC – Airway, Breathing, Circulation – comes another C – control of the principal killer, catastrophic bleeding. The marine's body is a 'container' and they have to make good the fluid lost when an IED blew off the 'container's' legs. In the shuddering helicopter, shouting instructions and information over the din, the team members, bulky with the clobber all soldiers wear under fire, insert lines into flat blood vessels. And I, as a new house officer, worried whether I could get an intravenous line into a patient I was escorting on the night train from Truro to London!

The technical skills of the army paramedics are impressive. So is the fact that they never forget that the 'container' is a fellow human being. They communicate with him gently, letting him know that they are with him also in spirit.

Despite the high-tech equipment, the tourniquet remains a vital tool. It was invented by a Frenchman and first employed in 1674. Its use is still debated, but the consensus is that though it may threaten some limbs it saves more lives. Soldiers can see that and some go into battle with tourniquets in place on each limb so they can tighten them without help if they are hit.

Vaughan Smith was 'embedded' with a US Army aviation

regiment. 'Embedding' enables journalists to get near the front line, though under circumstances which restrict what they can report. It's a trade-off, but Smith was able to convey the reality of what the medics are doing. Not just for the injured soldiers. They evacuate civilians, even enemy Taliban, if they need it. There is no escaping the human cost of war .

Military medicine has become more effective over the centuries, often despite those in command of armies. Wellington may have beaten the French on the battlefield but it was Napoleon who thought injured solders' lives were worth saving. Stretchers were introduced to remove the French wounded promptly from the battlefield. Fifty years later the British generals in the Crimea didn't think stretchers worth unloading from the troopships. And though most armies now commit to care for wounded combatants, medicine has struggled to keep up with the technology of killing.

One thing that has never changed is the courage of the medics. They used to work behind the lines, which was dangerous enough. In 21st-century conflicts everywhere is a front line, and, as Vaughan Smith's video shows, the medics pick up the wounded from the heart of the fighting. The nearer the medics are to the battle, the more wounded soldiers survive, but the greater the risk to highly trained personnel whose skills are literally vital.

Not many soldiers go to war to save lives. Army medics do. Increasingly successfully, as the survival statistics show. One in four soldiers seriously injured in combat in Vietnam died; in Afghanistan it is around one in fourteen. This has raised the question of whether the medivac units should be considered a 'force multiplier'. Under the Geneva Convention, vehicles bearing a red cross enjoy safe passage. But if they make the force significantly more effective, they could be regarded as increasing the strength of the army. It isn't that those extra ten lives saved mean ten soldiers return to combat. Most are too seriously injured ever to go to war again. But because the soldiers know they are going to be looked after, the effect on morale is substantial. Would the Taliban be justified in shooting at the medivac helicopters? Should the tourniquet be considered an offensive weapon? War is hell, but we are still working out the rules for civilised behaviour in hell.

Blood and Dust *can be seen on www.journalism.co.uk or YouTube*

—NASGP April 2011

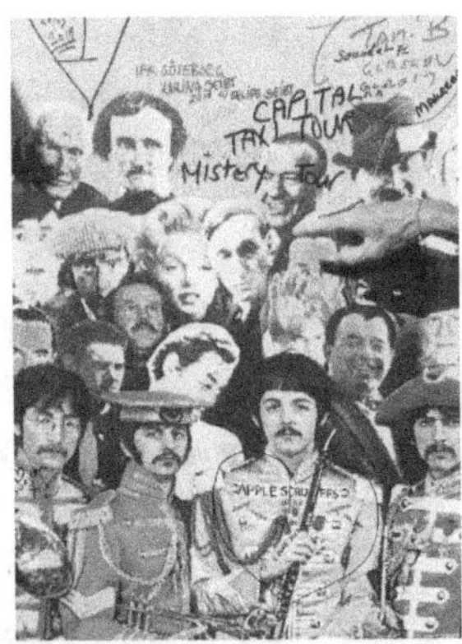

Medicine Needs Mavericks

When eminent hospital consultants write their memoirs they are not just summing up their careers, they reflect on the changes they have lived through. And when they are retired, they can say what they think.

Neurosurgeon Henry Marsh set the trend with *Do No Harm*. Stephen Westaby, in *Fragile Lives*, tells how a lad from a council estate in Scunthorpe became a cardiac surgeon whose expertise was such that colleagues summoned him back from Australia to operate on a case they felt no-one else could tackle. From him I learned how 'ventricular assist devices' can tide patients over till their own heart heals or a transplant becomes available. And that patients given Jarvik artificial hearts are surviving as long as transplant patients do. And that they have no pulse – a trap for unwary first-responders.

Urology has fewer life-and-death dramas, but like his fellow memoirists, Gautam Das puts the reader in his theatre clogs. In *Tender Is the Scalpel's Edge*, he reminds us that the skills and judgement of the surgeon must be backed up by an experienced and dedicated team. Like his colleagues, he ponders how you give a patient a realistic picture of a grim future without destroying hope, even of a few more days of life.

Neurology can't compete with the high-wire glamour of surgery. Patients may have intellectually fascinating diseases, but there are few happy ends: effective treatments are in short supply and cures are non-existent.

In his memoir, Andrew Lees reviews his career as a world expert in Parkinson's Disease. Like Westaby he explores new treatments. Like Marsh his subject is the brain. Marsh wonders how the grey jelly on which he operates can generate consciousness. Lees can only help his patients if he can modify the brain's neuronal activity.

How do you unravel the relationship of structure to function in an organ which has 100 billion neurons, 100 trillion synapses and hundreds of transmitters?

We have barely begun. Dopamine wasn't identified in the brain till 1955, and only in 1960 was it recognised that it is deficient in people with Parkinson's. In the mid-60s the first trials of L-dopa treatment changed patients' lives. But the shine wore off the miracle when patients developed motor complications. Research was decades from generating effective new therapies. Yet there are people with plenty of experience of the effects of chemicals on the brain. Lees turned to William Burroughs. And called his memoir *Mentored by a Madman*.

A middle-class American medical school drop-out, Burroughs joined the Beat Generation and spent his life testing the effect of all the mind-altering drugs he could get hold of, and recording their effects. The truth of his life is barely less extraordinary than his fiction. The Beatles included him in *Sgt. Pepper's Lonely Hearts Club Band*.

When Lees was a disillusioned medical student he came across *Naked Lunch*, Burroughs' semi-autobiographical sex-and-drugs-and-degradation counterculture novel. His interest in Burroughs was reawakened by Oliver Sacks' unorthodox treatment of patients with encephalitis lethargica, described in *Awakenings*.

Lees reasoned that if the drugs Burroughs took evoked or mitigated either Parkinsonian symptoms or the side effects of L-dopa, might they not be pointers to compounds with therapeutic applications? Ergot has a structure related to dopamine. Forty thousand patients had been treated with LSD, an ergot derivative, for alcoholism and mental disorders, with encouraging results, until 1966 when politics relegated LSD back to counterculture use. Lees investigated other, related, compounds. How about apomorphine, which Burroughs, and later Keith Richards, found the only effective treatment for opioid addiction? How about amphetamines? Or yagé, the hallucinogen sacred to Amazonian shamans?

Lees' detective work takes him through a maze which twists and turns and leads up blind alleys and loops back on itself. He analyses the experiences of the self-experimenters for clues. He questions received opinion. He tries compounds on himself. At the age of 66, this eminent professor at Queen Square follows

Burroughs' footsteps to the Amazon, the source of so many hallucinogens, to experience for himself the effects of yagé, and be blown away.

The highs, the lows and the frustrations of Lees' search for treatments for Parkinson's echo Westaby's experiences in his work on artificial hearts. The NHS has become risk averse. But you cannot wait for a committee to approve the management of an intraoperative crisis. You cannot start large-scale trials until small-scale observational work has suggested a hypothesis to test. And as the story of marijuana for patients with MS shows, there is still huge sensitivity about trials of hallucinogenic drugs for therapeutic use.

Hospital authorities have their eye on mortality statistics and bottom lines. They question professionals' judgement. Innovation may be seen as a threat. They aim to control doctors, managing their activities to minimise risk. But they still can't tell a Stephen Westaby from a rogue doctor like Ian Paterson.

Sick patients see things differently. Patients in end-stage heart failure know they are dying. Patients locked up by severe Parkinson's exist in a living death. They have nothing to lose and are willing to take the chance that an experimental treatment may work. Should bureaucracy deny them an informed choice?

The sense of vocation which has propelled these doctors to give so much shines out of these memoirs. So does the stress: to be always available, to sacrifice marriages and family life and sometimes health. They hear politicians being dishonest about the capabilities and funding of the NHS, and denigrating doctors. They see managers who appear to be more concerned about dress codes than patients. They all worry that the commitment and training of young doctors is being eroded by 21st-century ambitions, shift work and the end of anything like apprenticeship.

When medicine is just another job and doctors are no longer professionals but cogs in a big corporate machine, they, patients and society – all of us – will be the poorer.

📖 ***Do No Harm: Stories of Life, Death and Brain Surgery***
Henry Marsh, 2014

📖 ***Fragile Lives: A Heart Surgeon's Stories of Life and Death on the Operating Table*** *Stephen Westaby, 2017*

📖 ***Tender Is the Scalpel's Edge: Stories from the Journal of an NHS Consultant Surgeon*** *Gautam Das, 2016*

📖 ***Mentored by a Madman: The William Burroughs Experiment***
Andrew Lees, 2016

SEE ALSO

📖 ***Admissions: A Life in Brain Surgery*** *Henry Marsh, 2017. Marsh looks to the future, and does not like what he foresees.*

📖 ***When Breath Becomes Air*** *Paul Kalanithi, 2017. Neurosurgeon Paul Kalanithi wrote his memoir in the months before he died of cancer at the age of 37.*

—NASGP June 2017

Photo: William Burroughs appeared as a member of 'Sgt. Pepper's Lonely Hearts Club Band', on the album cover shown here painted on the wall of the EMI studio in St John's Wood, London, on the occasion of the 50th anniversary of the recording made there.

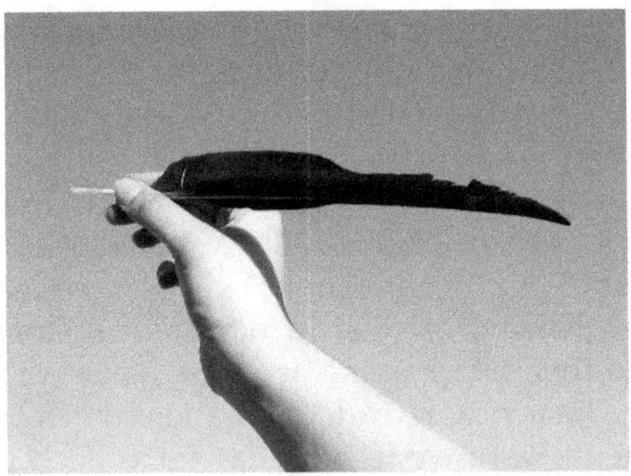

Why Doctors Should Write Poems

Hilton Koppe is a genial Australian GP whose talent for engaging an audience can be judged by the fact that he can cajole Aussie orthopods to write poetry. His thesis is that we spend our lives writing down patients' stories, but are not encouraged to reflect on them or allowed to admit our emotional involvement. He argues that we need a way of making sense of the dramas which we witness, and creative writing offers us that opportunity.

At this year's conference in Basel of the World Organisation of Family Doctors, Dr Koppe persuaded a multinational audience of GPs to choose their most memorable heartsink patient and to write down adjectives beginning with B to describe them. Aussies apparently are good at this: 'b****y crazy', 'b****y maddening', 'b****y pain in the a**e'. We were then given a simple verse structure – no rhymes required – and ten minutes to write about our chosen patient. Several participants responded to the invitation to read out their work. Most wrote in English, for many their second or third language. One participant explained that he thought that AU against Dr Koppe's name in the conference timetable meant 'Austrian', and had he realised that the workshop was being run by an Australian he, a Kiwi, would have joined the session on teenage health in Slovenia. Still, he read out his poem. A GP from Basel explained that she had written in her mother tongue, but was confident we would understand. We did. Few languages can express frustration as satisfyingly as *Schweizerdeutsch*.

We then moved on to consider some event in the past that rankled still. Easy. My first surgical firm as a medical student. Had I not given up so much to go to medical school, I might well have quit training at that point, so negative was the model presented to me of the profession I was struggling to join. Dr Koppe asked us to write in prose without stopping to think, just letting the words flow. I was amazed at the bitterness which poured from my pen. We then had to write from the point of view of the other side. For me, that meant the surgery tutor who declined to teach because it was "spoon-feeding". The exercise was enlightening. And therapeutic.

There is a growing interest in narrative – story-telling – in medicine. And this is happening at a time when we are losing the richness of the historical record. Old patient notes are fascinating social documents, as anyone who has gone back through thick Lloyd George envelopes knows. When they are shredded so is much of our history. Doctors don't write like that nowadays. Not just because patients now have the right to read what we write. What renders 21st-century records so sterile is the medico-legal sword of Damocles. So the kernel of the patient's story is lost in a thicket of possibly significant negatives. Gone are the days when a doctor conjured up a patient by writing "there she sits at the bar looking like Marilyn Monroe but twice as vulnerable".

GPs are witnesses to events which challenge people's lives. Perhaps as we leach emotional colour from the medical records we have more need to find outlets for our feelings about the stories in which we play this strange role. Try poetry.

My poem, the first I've ever written, was about my heartsink patient, 'Annie':

Who's shaking whom?
Get it together, Annie,
Get a grip.
Get a life.
Get away.
Get a pair of boots and start walking.
Do all this before I get my gun.

—NASGP October 2009

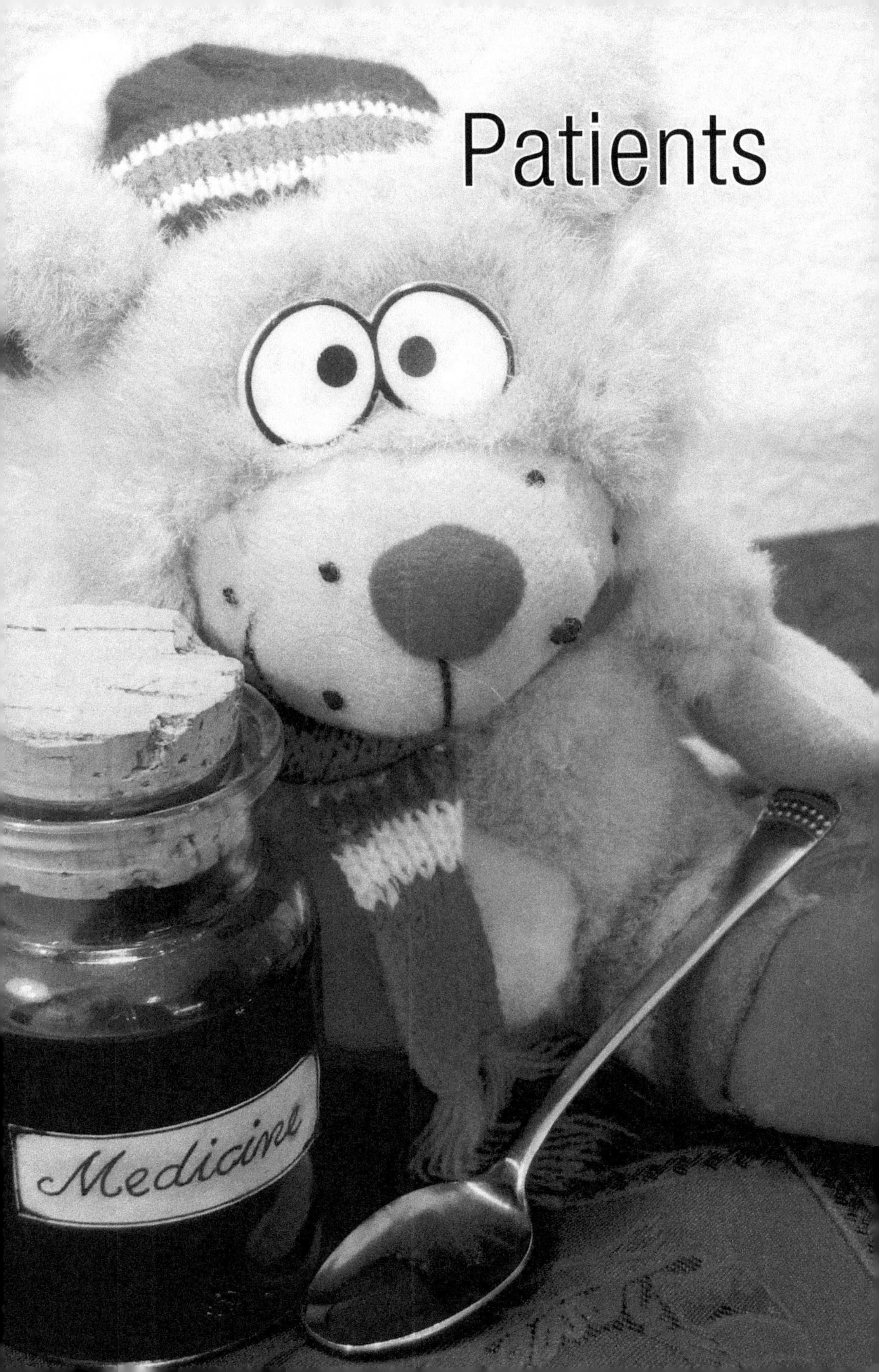

Patients
Medicine

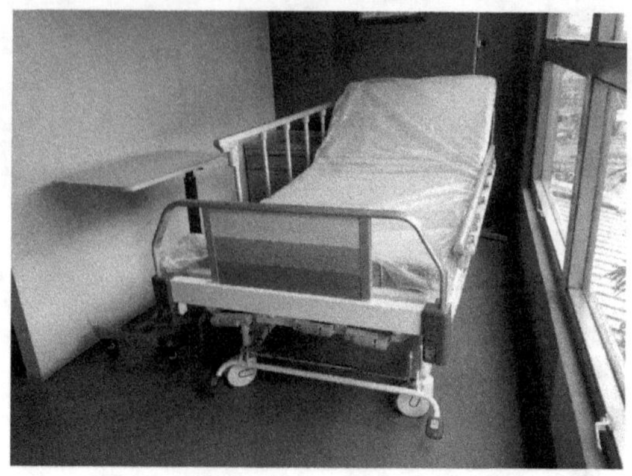

Sleeping with the Patient

Mrs M was the patient. She might or might not have been dementing, but she seemed confused and was certainly prone to wandering. She might or might not have been in severe pain from her arthritis, but she certainly had a flail leg after failed surgery. All of which made it difficult for her to live in her isolated cottage with its steep narrow staircase. Somehow her medication had reached alarming levels and might or might not have been making things worse. She was in the cottage hospital for evaluation. Essentially this meant taking her off her psychotropics and titrating her pain relief. After several days no-one was sure what was going on. Does paracetamol take effect within half a minute? Was she skipping down the corridor when she thought no-one was watching? Was she attention-seeking? She was certainly much more peaceful when someone spent time with her.

I was in my GP trainee year, and on call. The previous evening the cottage hospital had not been busy and the nursing staff had popped in regularly to see Mrs M. Everyone had had a quiet night. Tonight the staff were occupied with a dying patient. At intervals through the evening they rang to say that Mrs M kept struggling out of bed and falling, and asking what could be done. In line with the agreed plan, I authorised further doses of major tranquilliser as I went from visit to visit.

Some time after midnight things quietened down, and I went to the cottage hospital to see how they were getting on. Badly. Mrs M was still creating problems the staff could not manage. I had no confidence that yet more medication would help. I could see no hope of going home to an undisturbed night. Mrs M was the only patient in a two-bedded room. After some thought, I asked the nurses to move her bed against the wall, and then we pushed the second bed alongside it. I got in and put my arm around Mrs M. There we lay until dawn, in uneasy repose. Every so often she would make a play for escape off the end of the bed and I would persuade her to lie down again.

Next afternoon, the psycho-geriatrician came to assess her. Standing on the steps of the cottage hospital chatting to a colleague before going in to hear his verdict, I noticed the door being pushed open. A familiar figure sidled around it, coat over her nightdress and slippers on her feet. I steered her back inside. "It's all very well for you; you can escape", she muttered. I could; she, on the other hand, disappeared into the psychogeriatric unit and from my life.

So I have spent a night in bed with a patient. It was unorthodox but not improper, and it solved the problem. Even with the hindsight of 18 years' more experience I don't have an alternative strategy.

—*NASGP May 2007*

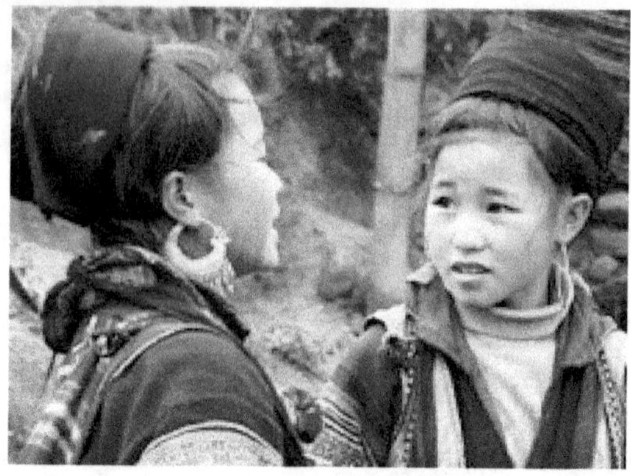

The Spirit Catches You and You Fall Down

During its war in Vietnam, the USA fought a secret action against the communists in Laos. The CIA recruited the aid of the Hmong, one of Indochina's hill tribes with little love for the Pathet Lao. Their participation cost the Hmong their lands and livelihoods, and many took advantage of American promises of reward in the USA. Few found their dreams fulfilled. The Lee family settled in Merced, a small city in California, with poor accommodation and few prospects. Their daughter Lia developed intractable epilepsy. *The Spirit Catches You and You Fall Down* is a compelling account of their engagement with the US health services.

Every A&E department has its heartsink patients; Lia, taken to the emergency room countless times in status epilepticus, was Merced hospital's heartsink. Hmong shamans rationalise epilepsy as what happens when the soul flies from the body: the spirit catches you and you fall down. Her parents were desperate to reunite their daughter's body and soul; her doctors were equally anxious to control her seizures. Lia's tragedy was that, try though they might, they could not find a way to do so.

The family wanted the help of conventional medicine. The paediatricians – an idealistic husband and wife team – were immensely caring and tried their best. But different social customs, lack of understanding, lack of a shared language, poor education, inflexibility – all created a gap which Lia slipped through.

The core of the problem – or perhaps what we would regard as the core of the problem – was Lia's medication. Lia's doctors did not want her to have second-rate treatment simply because she was from a disadvantaged immigrant community, so they strove to develop a perfect regime. The trouble was that the family could not understand the complex and continually changing medication schedule, and all they saw was that the medicines were making their daughter ill. Finally, Lia was fit-free, but at a terrible cost.

Could it happen here? Lia's doctors saw second-best as a form of prejudice. In the underfunded NHS we are used to muddle and compromise. We accept that people may be illiterate, that they may not know their date of birth or immunisation status, and that their family structures are different from ours. British GP training is about understanding the patient's point of view and negotiating a mutually acceptable management plan.

But we should not feel smug. Last week I saw a middle-aged Somali woman. She looked twenty years older than her age. She had consulted many times about her pain, often as an emergency with no interpreter. Many things had been tried. She was no better, her daughter told me while her mother leaned back in the chair, her eyes closed, groaning and rubbing her side. Her mother felt that we didn't care. I suspect my patient's views and those of Lia's parents would have been similar, and that my frustration would have echoed that felt by the doctors in Merced.

It has recently been suggested that the NHS should stop funding interpreters on the grounds that immigrants would then be forced to learn English. The idea that axing interpreter services will encourage integration seems ludicrous. Once you are over the age of ten, it takes quite a time to become fluent enough in a language to negotiate another country's bureaucracy. If you are elderly it usually takes more effort than you are able to make — ask the Brits who retire to the Costa del Sol. Without interpreters social equity is impossible. Unless someone explains, how can you understand the practice's appointment system? Or the NHS referral system – something that does not exist in countries where direct access to specialists is the norm? How can you understand about pills and potions and side effects? And how can I understand what you are feeling, and how you interpret your symptoms and what you fear? I suspect that the kindness of doctors is for many immigrants their first encounter with humanity in the UK. We have a crucial role in helping people feel that Britain is a good place to be and we need to make the most of it.

📖 *The Spirit Catches You and You Fall Down* Anne Fadiman, 1998

—NASGP August 2008

Photo: Hmong women in Sapa, Vietnam

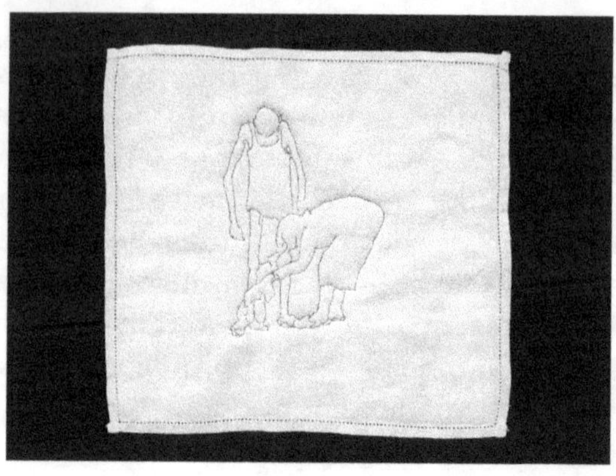

Drawing Dementia

With a few lines on a piece of paper Hans Holbein created pictures which 500 years later still convey the characters of living people. I wouldn't have dreamed that it was possible to achieve that with a sewing machine. But Georgie Meadows can do it. The inspiration for her *Stitched Drawings* comes from her work as an occupational therapist with elderly people with dementia. She says she doesn't feel she has total control over a picture: it's a bit like dementia: a sewn line shows a forlorn old man's sagging shoulders. Loose threads illustrate the disordered hair of an old lady. Another elderly lady struggles to get a pair of trousers up her husband's spindly legs.

Most of us fear dementia, for our families and friends, and for ourselves. As doctors many of us find patients with dementia difficult – they are hard to communicate with, hard to warm to, hard to help. But even if we escape the shadow of dementia in our personal lives, it is our job and will be an increasing burden to our ageing society.

It is difficult enough to remember that people with dementia still have something to offer us, the able-brained, let alone to know how to reach it. So much of modern everyday life calls for the capabilities which dementia takes away, and most of us are better at helping people with worn-out knees than worn-out brains.

Georgie Meadows' drawings evoke our compassionate instincts. And she has found a way to harness the urge to help. Go to Monmouth on Thursday afternoons and join her weekly Tea Dance. Many people at the tea dances have dementia, but far from all. Elderly people who are lonely, housewives looking for social exercise, teenagers, children, anyone is welcome. As the short film, *Thursday Afternoons*, which accompanies her exhibition, shows, everyone is enjoying themselves. People whose brains fail them when asked about what they had for breakfast remember the dances they learned when they were young. Some can even pick up new steps.

And dancing means physical contact. If you haven't had a hug for years, what could be nicer than to foxtrot round the floor in someone's arms – arms which offer support so the tottery don't fall. And even in a wheelchair you can still dance with your arms.

Visiting a dementing relative in a care home can be grim. How much better to accompany granny to the tea dance and see her come alive again, for youngsters to find she isn't so frightening, for middle-aged sons and daughters to realise that they and their frail parent can still share pleasures.

Singing, like dancing, is a rewarding social activity which calls on patterns of behaviour laid down in our deep memory banks. Play the *Hallelujah Chorus* in a care home and a surprising number of residents will be roused from their twilight world to join in. Or try them with *The White Cliffs of Dover*. Or *Yellow Submarine*. 'Singing for the Brain' is an Alzheimer's Society initiative which does with singing what Georgie Meadows does with dancing. And drawing can unlock memories, too. But these days schools don't demand rote learning. Will we have fewer memories to draw on when we need them?

Dementia cafes, another venture to provide normal, social activities for people with dementia and for their carers, and a source of advice, help and support for all, started in UK in Farnborough in 2000. Now there is probably one near you.

Physical activity, music, shared experiences, make us all feel calmer, less anxious, more in control. They relieve boredom and give us a place in the community. So it seems common sense that people with dementia should benefit, though no studies have yet been done to prove it. But activities need to be the intellectual equivalent of tai chi: looking for what the person can still do rather than demoralising them by exposing what they can't. As Georgie Meadows points out, routine and continuity are important. People and events which come and go just make confusion worse. The Monmouth Tea Dances have been a regular fixture since 2006.

No-one pretends that these ventures are the whole answer to the increasing burden of dementia. But they may mitigate, at least somewhat, the pitiful wailing and the awful restlessness of the old lady in the corner of the care home lounge. A different model is a purpose-built village for people with dementia, with staff playing the role of shopkeepers, publicans, hairdressers. There are dementia villages in Holland and Switzerland. You may object to the deceit, but people who live in 'Dementiaville' seem a lot happier than those confined to the average home for the elderly mentally infirm.

Can a million people be trained into friendship? Last month, the government and Alzheimer's Society, launched a campaign to recruit that number of Dementia Friends. My first reaction was to shrink from the idea of manufacturing emotion. Is mass awareness really going to make a difference? It won't help the severely affected; they need professional care. But Dementia Friends has worked in Japan. An elderly man at Tesco's checkout is searching helplessly for – he doesn't remember what. If the cashier can recognise that he probably has early dementia, and knows how to help him, and how to deal with impatient customers in the queue, she will be helping everyone.

If dementia gets you down, look at Georgie Meadows' stitched drawings on her website www.georgiemeadows.co.uk. They will restore your compassion.

Thursday Afternoons *is available on www.cromwellfilms.com*

—NASGP December 2012

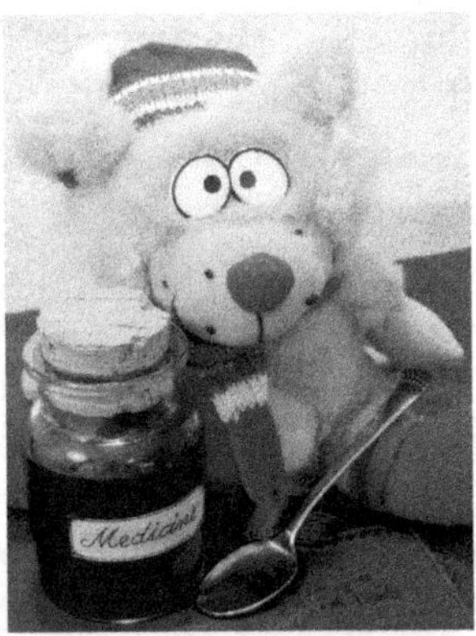

Get Well Soon!

"When I go into hospital for an operation, I always re-read *Ulysses*." I would have taken the speaker as a resident of 'Pseud's Corner' until I remembered that after a high-impact landing on my left shoulder brought a skiing holiday to an abrupt end, I read *Ulysses*. Well, it was that or Danielle Steel in German.

But passing time while you are condemned to the sick role but not actually feeling unwell is very different from being properly ill. Could anybody in bed with flu manage to get through *Ulysses*? That would be a diagnostic test, like dropping a £20 banknote on the floor and checking whether the patient gets out of bed to pick it up. If you can, you haven't got flu.

So what helps the sick recover? A good story, heavy enough not to feel that your brain is rotting but light enough to be held by weak hands and enjoyed by a fuzzy brain, certainly. Long books to while away the long hours seem a good idea. Perhaps *War and Peace*, an involving tale with a huge cast of characters, and it comes in two easy-to-manage volumes. But it is 1,500 pages. If somebody gives it to you as a patient, do they know something you don't?

Surroundings are important. Research has confirmed what we all know intuitively: patients get better faster if they can see trees from their sickbed. Unfortunately the outlook from most old city hospital wards is Victorian industrial grime or 1960s stained concrete. Hospitals built during the Second World War were designed with plenty of space to reduce the risk of an enemy bomb demolishing the whole facility, but by now the green spaces have been filled in with car parks and Portacabins. Modern hospital design tends to the vertical. Recently I visited a 10th floor ward. One bay had an uninterrupted view of the weather, always changing, always interesting. However, the other bay looked out on two nearby office blocks, attractive enough in a Richard Rogers-lite way when seen from a distance, but angular and uncomfortable seen from close range.

Most hospitals have realised there is money to be made from providing distraction from the inevitably mildly depressing reality of a hospital ward. If the cricket is essential to your wellbeing or the suspense of waiting for the next episode of *Emmerdale* is bad for your heart, the price demanded for plugging into the bedside entertainment system may be worth paying. Some channels may be free – radio, for example, although why can you listen to Radio 4 and Classic FM but not Radio 3? Who makes these decisions?

The healing properties of art are well known, though outside of outpatient departments, patients rarely get to see it. Yet it can benefit the health of other hospital residents: in my SHO days the row of original prints along the long corridor of a hospital nourished my spirit as I staggered down to see yet another ?MI at 3 a.m. It's a shame that the view from most hospital beds is the intimidating battery of apparatus on the wall behind the bed of the patient opposite. A tangle of coloured tubing and cabling might suggest a painting by Joan Miró, though he's perhaps not the most therapeutic of artists.

Visitors are a welcome distraction, but making the visit a healing pleasure rather than a trying duty can be hard. The geography of the bed, the drip stands, the table and chairs makes impossible the comfortable intimacy of home or even of the counsellor's consulting room. You can't easily share a crossword or even the cricket. In the hubbub of the ward companionable silence is very difficult, a chaste but comforting cuddle almost impossible.

The reality is that if you are in hospital, you are in hospital, and classy curtaining and Monet prints will not disguise even a private room. Better entertainment, good food and a pleasant outlook help. Having visitors when you are in hospital is like having visitors when you are in prison. They are welcome and valued, and they may even be able to smuggle in a treat or two, but the situation is still abnormal. What really makes a difference is the staff. When you are sitting there waiting for a theatre slot to become vacant or for the drip to finish, a smile is the best thing that can happen to you. It lifts the spirits, it eases pain and fear, it makes you feel part of the human race. When I think back to my days as a hospital doctor, I just hope I smiled.

—*NASGP October 2009*

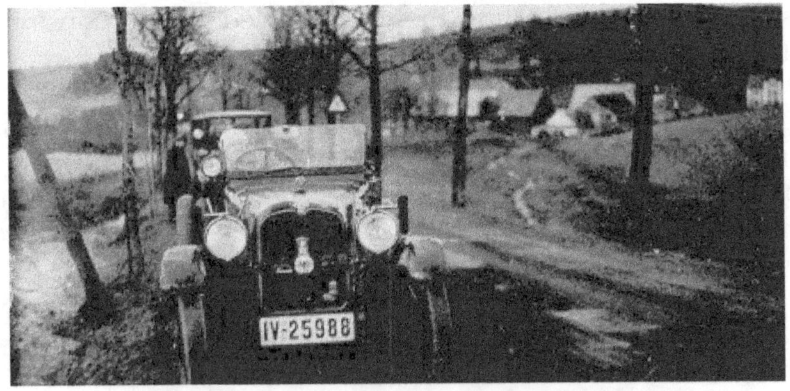

Can You See the STOP Sign?

"My 85-year-old father isn't safe to drive any longer, but he absolutely refuses to stop." It's a common theme round the dinner table. And in the consulting room too, where exasperated families come hoping the GP can 'do something'. But there isn't much we can do. We can be firm with patients, we may be asked by the DVLA to perform a simple health check, and we can contact the DVLA if we feel that the public good justifies it, but we rarely have experience of our patients' driving skills. "I would be happy to sit beside you driving" a GP told an elderly driver I know well. I have been her passenger. Clearly he never has. And discussing driving ability can be the end of the doctor-patient relationship. Tell a patient that they have a terminal illness and they will probably be distressed and frightened; tell them they shouldn't be driving and the response is denial and anger.

The DVLA requires elderly drivers to fill in a long form before it will renew their licences, and may require an independent eye check. Unlike many public examinations which require an acceptable average mark over every element, your driving licence will be renewed if you scrape a pass on the visual test. No-one checks that you can compensate for only-just-adequate vision through good reflexes, concentration, mental processing, and judgement. And what about hearing? And stiff necks? You need to be able to turn your head easily to look around you. And how many 85-year-olds have the physical strength to manage a powerful BMW in an emergency? Plus, you need road sense. Elderly drivers often choose inappropriate speeds, shooting onto roundabouts and crawling along motorways. Some interpret street signs and rights of way creatively, claiming that because the instructions are 'misleading' they are absolved from responsibility. Yet there is no assessment of road sense.

Ophthalmologists can be over-generous, for instance giving a 90-year-old permission to drive on condition that he stays at home after dark. The driver had to take his wife to hospital. It wasn't till 10 p.m. that she was settled and he felt free to start the familiar 20-minute drive home. Three hours later two police cars had to escort him to his front door.

It takes obstinacy and independence to be driving at 95. Not qualities which predispose drivers to trade in their car for Dial-A-Ride after decades behind the wheel. "I've never had an accident", many say. But their cars clearly have. "I only drive locally and these days I go very slowly." But over-80s have more accidents per mile than any other drivers.

How do the elderly come to realise that their driving days are over? A small but dangerous misjudgement may frighten them into exchanging the car for a taxi. Some find a face-saving way of giving up. My aunt lost, or 'lost', her car keys. Others accept proffered lifts because "it's not a nice day to be driving", and somehow it never is 'nice enough' to drive. But with a worryingly high number, pleading, financial arguments, logic, elaboration of the risks of driving and information about the alternatives fall on deaf ears. If you feel that your life is not worth living without a car, even the argument that your driving could end someone else's life carries no weight.

The baby-boomers will be coming up to 80 in the next decade or so. What should we be doing to remove from our roads a large and vociferous cohort of elderly drivers who are convinced they are safe drivers when they're not? If their children disconnect the battery or let down the tyres the parent will just call the AA. Driving for many elderly people is not just a pleasure but a symbol of independence: "It's my lifeline". Arguing that using a car to go to the shops is just a convenience or a habit misses the point. It *is* a lifeline, but to a sense of self-worth. For many, relinquishing their licence is relinquishing living. No subsidised taxi scheme can compensate for that. How can we persuade our elderly relatives, friends and patients, and, in years to come, ourselves, that we can be independent and valued even when we no longer hold the car keys?

It is easier to be obliged by an inflexible rule to give up than to admit that you aren't the person you were. So maybe no-one over the age of, say, 85, should be licensed to drive? Or should we have a more comprehensive assessment of all the faculties everyone needs to be a safe driver? In Spain elderly drivers are required to play a videogame, steering an electronic car along a winding road. What a good screening test for reflexes and judgement! Why don't we make a driving simulator test mandatory for all people applying for a renewal of their licence? Any other ideas?

—*NASGP December 2010*

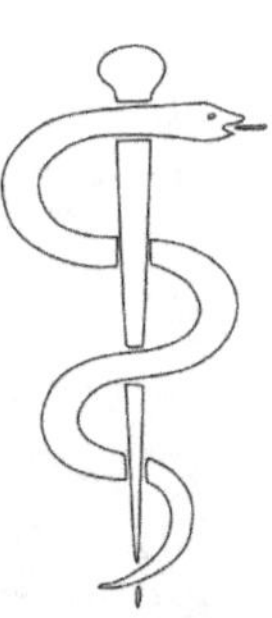

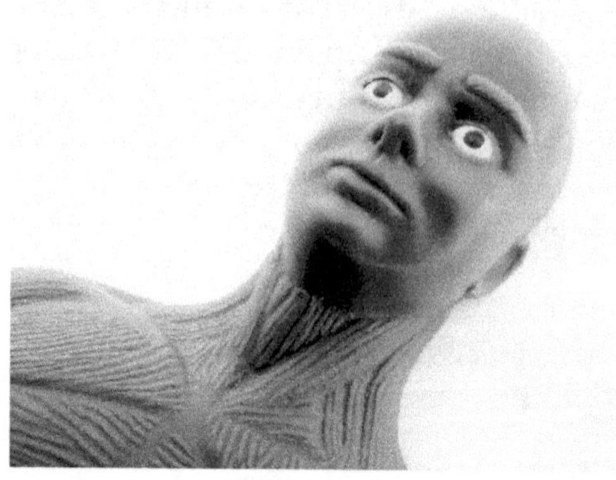

The Trouble with Dennis

Dennis was in the fourth bed on the left. When I joined the firm he had already been there some while. Every ward round, the collective morale of the team would sink when we came to his bed. After weeks we still didn't know what was wrong with him. From his pillow, Dennis regarded us with truculent challenge.

Every week his long frame was a little thinner, his look a little more withering. He seemed to be willing himself to deny us the satisfaction of a diagnosis and the reward of seeing him recover.

One afternoon the cardiac arrest bleep went off. Fourth bed on the left.

We were uncomfortable. We didn't know what he had died of. His family didn't seem that bothered, but we were. A post-mortem was agreed. But the mortuary technician was in Benidorm and the hospital couldn't do any autopsies. The pathologist at St Elsewhere's would perform a coroner's post-mortem and provide specimens for his colleague at our hospital.

As the junior member of the team, I was chosen to attend the post-mortem and transport the specimens. The pathologist at St Elsewhere's gave a jolly running commentary. He sliced chunks off various organs and offered them to me with the flourish of a waiter at a carvery. With a sweet jar full of bits of my former patient, I set off on the return journey. The roads were busy, the day was hot, the formalin was leaking from the jar. If I were stopped by the police, would they believe me? If I had an accident, how would I explain? "Don't worry," the SHO had said, "I'm sure they will be able to tell which bits are you and which are Dennis."

We reached home, I in one piece and Dennis in a dozen. The pathologist's report, when it came, was not enlightening. It told us some things we knew and nothing that we did not know. We still had no insight into what Dennis had lived with and died of.

I have come to terms with not knowing how Dennis died. Medicine is not an exact science. Though 21st-century imaging, 20th-century biochemistry and 19th-century pathology can shed light on many conundrums, none is guaranteed to provide all the answers. Knowing as much as we do, it may be harder for us to accept being denied knowledge, but if we are wise we accept that sometimes we are not going to know. Primitive people can wish themselves to death, and we recognise the part the psyche plays in the time and manner of death in many patients in our technological world. Whether Dennis willed his own demise and whether he wanted to humble us, I cannot know. But remembering that unsettling journey with the sweet jar, I can hear Dennis laughing the last laugh.

—*NASGP October 2010*

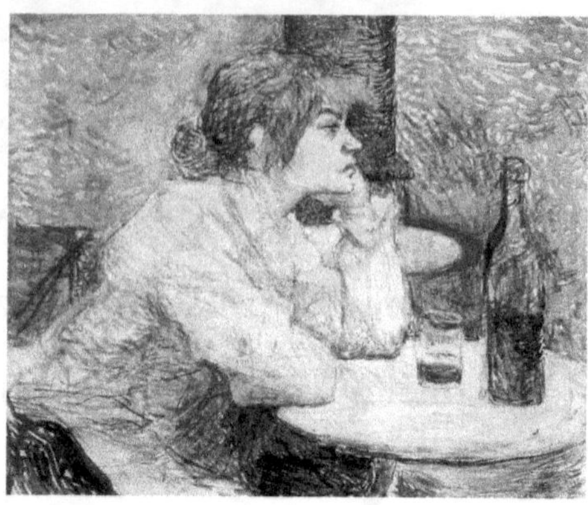

Facing Up to the Demon

"You could try AA, but they're a funny lot. And you alcoholics tend to be a clever bunch . . ." So said the counsellor my friend was seeing about her problem drinking. She was flattered: "Oh, how we alcoholics love to be told that we're extra-clever!" Alcoholics Anonymous, it seemed, was cultish, prescriptive, quite possibly exploitative, and clearly to be avoided. It was another four years before she overcame her prejudices, went to AA, and found a way out of drinking.

Like many GPs, I didn't encourage patients to go to AA, and I wonder how many lives we condemn as a consequence. Most organisations dealing with alcohol problems are run by professionals whose approach we understand. For us, AA doesn't fit in the box. A bunch of recovering drunks helping other drunks? Can you imagine the patient who sits by the war memorial with cans of Tennent's Super standing up to say "I am Pete and I am an alcoholic"? The businessman saying "I am Simon and I am an alcoholic"? What about the religiosity of AA's 'Twelve Steps' programme? It's not going to work.

But it does. Talking to people who have quit drinking through AA has opened my eyes, and if this article sounds like an advertisement, it's because I think we fail our patients if we don't give them a realistic picture of an organisation which might be the answer for them. AA works. Not for everyone, of course, and there have been no controlled trials, but many people can testify to its efficacy.

What drives people to AA? When my friend faced the humiliation of being too drunk to take part in the lunch party she had organised, she was desperate enough to take that first step and admit that she could not control her drinking. Others reached the turning point less dramatically, but all eventually recognised that they were on a one-way trip to an ignominious death. They describe walking into their first meeting unable to stop drinking and walking out at the end feeling that they had a choice.

A few facts. AA takes the view that for alcoholics, drink has become a mental obsession and a physical compulsion. Alcoholics, like those with severe allergies, are only safe if they forswear the substance which harms them. So, like most agencies dealing with addiction, AA would answer the patient who asked me "Can't I be a part-time alcoholic?" with a resounding "No".

Thousands of meetings take place every day, organised by the members themselves. AA receives no subsidies but membership is free. Those who can, contribute to the costs of hiring the venue.

AA is always there. Many alcoholics ask doctors for immediate help, but few organisations are able to see them there and then. It is said that the waiting tests the alcoholic's commitment. Is that a rationalisation of our inability to provide a same-day appointment with an alcohol service? So, are we missing the window of opportunity to address their problem? In towns there are often several AA meetings a week; in cities there will be meetings every day. One alcoholic remembers his GP printing off the list of local AA meetings. He went along that evening and has been dry ever since. And he still attends regularly. "I'd been through all the usual agencies. I'd had all the advice. I still couldn't keep off the booze. At AA I found the understanding that only other alcoholics can offer. A new social environment gave me strength and it still does. It's like aftercare."

When you join a group you have to own up to your alcoholism, but since everyone there has had a drink problem, you are among peers. "For the first time in years, I had no need to lie." Of course, it isn't all plain sailing. My friend returned home from her first meeting to a domestic emergency. Waiting for the plumber, she wrestled with the voice in her head which told her that it was a crisis, and a drink in a crisis was OK. Surviving that hour was the start of her recovery.

Yes, AA does have a spiritual side, which everyone I talked to felt was the key to its success for them. It may be a paradox, but they find that their own powerlessness is redeemed by a higher power. For some, it is God, for others the group, or whatever image gives them the willpower to live without alcohol.

The 'aftercare' includes having a sponsor – someone with a

longer experience of abstinence, who acts as a counsellor – so members always have someone to help them find an alternative to reaching for a drink. Being a sponsor can be affirming. "For the first time for years I feel useful and valued." Milestones are celebrated. "I thought I would feel ridiculous, but the cake for my first anniversary made me feel special."

AA is worldwide. My friend, posted to Italy, continued to go to meetings. They helped her stay sober during a stressful year away from home, and what better way to meet local people and improve her Italian!

Some doctors know a lot about AA. Medicine is, after all, a profession with a high rate of alcoholism. Doctors may be anxious about encountering their patients if they join a local AA group. One doctor found the British Doctors and Dentists Group a good place to start, but now goes to AA as well. There seems to be an egalitarian acceptance and a security in AA groups which gives doctors the confidence to go down to the Saturday morning meeting in their local church hall. And even celebrities. On *Desert Island Discs* recently, footballer Tony Adams chose the *AA Big Book* to take to his island.

After listening to people talk about their experiences, it seems that AA is effective because it is different. But AA is not a cult. It does not demand that you surrender your worldly goods or your soul to the organisation. It doesn't demand separation from your family. In fact, the reverse. Looking inwards to the group, these alcoholics have gained the strength to look outwards and engage with the world again.

—NASGP August 2010

Photo: *The Drinker*, Henri de Toulouse-Lautrec, 1888, Harvard University

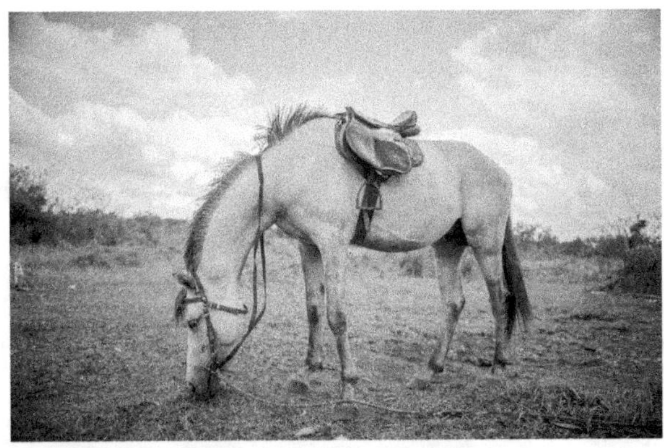

It's a Knockout!

If you had asked me about concussion a couple of months ago, I would probably have scratched my head and muttered about headaches. Now I am living with it, but I still find it hard to describe.

What led up to the concussion? I am dependent on the observations of others, because in effect I wasn't there. I remember riding up a leafy lane leading onto Dartmoor on a lovely late-September day. The next thing I recall is lying on a hospital trolley feeling a hard collar with holes in it around my neck, and being told that I had fallen off the horse and injured my head six hours ago, that I'd had a normal CT scan but was going to be kept in hospital overnight for observation. I recall the regular disturbance to have my blood pressure taken and a light shone in my eyes, the kind efficiency of the A&E staff, the NHS toast and tea next morning.

As we drove home, my husband told me what had happened. Nothing impressive: we had left the lane and were up on the moor, my horse was restive and started to canter, I lost a stirrup and slipped off. Not onto granite, onto a gorse bush. No obvious head injury, and yes, I was wearing a helmet, but there must have been enough of a wallop for me to be unconscious for several minutes and to have no memory of the fall (just as well if I were ever going to get on a horse again). I have no picture of being in the Land Rover, the drive over the moor to the cottage hospital, the ambulance trip to Exeter and the CT scan. During that time I had tried persistently to understand what had happened – asking endlessly where I was and why I was there. For a while I thought John Major was the Prime Minister, but by the time I reached the cottage hospital I am told I was able to recall the names of my current colleagues, though still perseverating with a litany of repetitive questions as I tried to anchor events in time and space.

For the first few days I couldn't read comfortably, or use a computer, and I couldn't bear music playing – it overloaded my brain. I didn't know that I try to deconstruct Bach fugues when I listen, but apparently so. I just slept. After a few days I picked up *A Short History of Tractors in the Ukraine*. Taken in short doses, just the thing for the bruised brain to practise on (those of you who haven't read it will be very puzzled).

After a couple of weeks I went back to practice for two days a week. I was safe enough – so much of what we do is embedded so deep that the blow had not shaken it out, and there are always people around should I get stuck. But for a while I was clumsy on the computer, and I am still slow. After a couple of sessions in which I ran 40 minutes late, I now have 20-minute appointments, a luxury both I and the patients will find it hard to relinquish.

Though the old knowledge is still intact and accessible, newer information tends to bob out of reach when I try to grasp it. Irregular Spanish subjunctives and QOF codes for example. And I haven't gone to any educational events; there doesn't seem any point in going through the ritual. Mental multitasking is still difficult, too. I am not up to driving round Camden on a wet, dark evening looking for blocks of flats. Could I cope if a patient were collapsed, or psychotic, or waving a knife at me? And I still tire easily and sleep badly – apparently a not uncommon sequel to a head injury.

Speaking to a neurologist was reassuring – six hours of amnesia is quite a long time compared with most knocks on the head, and, as they say in Cornwall, "the age is there", so I can expect it to take three months for my mental processing to return to its normal speed and complexity. And if I do too much I will only set myself back. I am learning that 'doing nothing' does not mean picking up the newspaper or fiddling on the computer. It means sitting with my eyes shut, doing . . . nothing.

I am told that during the hours of amnesia, I kept asking "Is this real?" For me, of course, it still isn't. No images have ever come back to fill in the black hole. I suppose that I realised that I was not forming memories. Neurologically, what processes were involved? When I am recovered I shall try and find out.

—*NASGP December 2006*

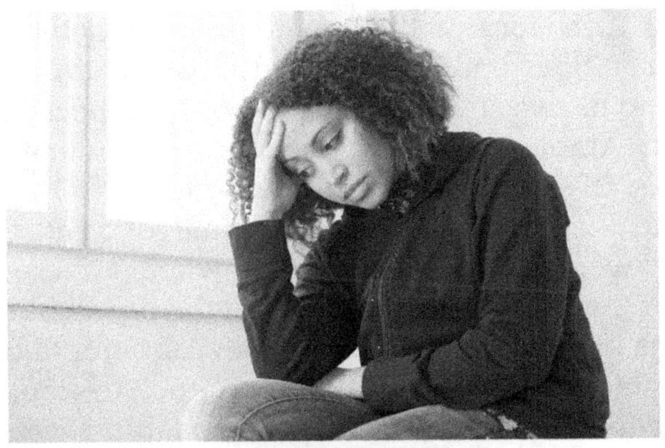

Bloody Hell!

You are 13 years old. Your family is poor. Each month you have to take a week off school. In a few months you are so behind in your school work that you drop out for ever. You live in an African country, in India, in the Australian outback . . . in Leeds.

You are 14 years old, and you live in a village in Nepal. Each month you are shut up in a hut for a week and left to yourself. It is cold. You light a fire and die of smoke asphyxiation.

You are a British teenager thrilled to be at Glastonbury. Your period comes on early. Your only pair of trousers is stained with the blood which is running down your legs. You wade through the mud to queue in the rain outside a toilet block. The vending machine is jammed with a counterfeit coin.

Throughout history menstruation has been regarded with suspicion. Bread made by menstruating women won't rise, crops will shrivel, men will be defiled by the evil eye. Prejudice is institutionalised. Menstruating women are feared and are sequestered from social and religious activities and from the marital bed till they are 'clean' again.

Since sanitary pads were introduced after the First World War, 'sanpro' has grown into an industry worth billions of dollars: a disposable product with a massive potential market. It could make life easier for half the world's population for 300 weeks of their existence. But poor women cannot afford it; only 10% of Indian women use sanitary protection. Worldwide, millions of women rely on rags or leaves or ashes or newspaper. These are ineffective, uncomfortable, they fall out, and they promote infections.

Decent sanitary protection provides dignity. It liberates women to complete their education, to work and socialise in confidence.

But only if their society, their menfolk, permit them access to information. A BBC reporter, being patted down on entry to Egypt, was found to have a strange object in her jeans pocket. What was it? Egyptian Arabic doesn't have the vocabulary to explain what a tampon is. Eventually, after all the tampons in the box in her luggage had been scanned, she was permitted to enter Egypt, and the security woman asked in a whisper whether these items were available in Cairo. Yes, in a few places, the reporter replied, and gave her the instruction leaflet. A small victory for liberation.

Programmes for donating sanitary products to schools, prisons, food banks (where they are more in demand than baked beans) and to the poor and homeless the world over are admirable, but they don't address all the problems and they aren't a sustainable solution. Also required are adequate water supplies, soap, privacy, disposal facilities and understanding. If you are transgender, unisex toilets may be helpful, but they make managing periods more difficult for another, much larger, section of society. And commercial products are made with plastic, and with cotton which requires huge quantities of water to grow. They take centuries to break down in landfill. They contain potentially irritant chemicals. They have to be distributed over long distances.

What is the answer? Reusable pads and silicone cups are catching on because women are spreading the word, but they can still be costly and they require cleaning and drying. In a close-knit society, who is going to hang out their pads to dry in the public gaze?

There are inspiring examples of locally made answers. Saathi, a woman-led company in Gujarat, makes disposable pads from banana fibres, a fully environmental and sustainable process. In Malawi, Trinitas Mhango Kunashe founded a social enterprise which makes reusable pads. In Tamil Nadu, Jayaashree Industries is the result of a five-year struggle by an uneducated villager to produce affordable sanitary protection. His wife, mother and society disowned him out of shame, but he finally invented a simple machine to make pads from local materials. It takes only three hours to learn to use it. Women's groups throughout India and beyond are buying it. It provides employment and dignity. I'm glad to say his wife returned to him and now supports the project.

Meanwhile, at home and abroad, women are bringing menstruation out of its discreet sanpro packaging and launching campaigns using social media. They use hashtags such as

#periodpositive and period-related emojis. It isn't easy: Ugandan activist Stella Nyanzi's campaign led to her imprisonment. President Trump's unpleasant misogynist tweets don't help – or are they so outrageous that they shock people into awareness? There are programmes to promote decent toilet facilities in educational establishments – I hope they have reached my former school.

Menstrual leave from work is contentious. Japan introduced it in 1947, and the idea has spread from the Far East to Italy and Bristol. But many women are too embarrassed to take advantage of it. And critics complain that it reinforces the view that women are unreliable employees. But in India, where periods are unmentionable, the heads of two companies have authorised menstrual leave and are making sure the press reports their action, to publicise the humiliating realities endured by Indian woman.

There is a very long way to go before menstruation is no longer a handicap. However many photos you post on Instagram of blood-stained white jeans and tampon threads, however right-on your sanitary protection, however liberated the men you work with are, there is no getting away from the fact that for many women periods are painful, messy, unpredictable and not a great topic of conversation, and pretending otherwise is to burden women with yet another guilt – that of failing to embrace menstruation in the correct spirit.

It is going to take time. It was Albert Einstein who said, "What a sad era when it is easier to smash an atom than a prejudice."

—NASGP August 2017

NEWSFLASH: Scotland has just become the first national government in the world to distribute free sanitary products to poor women through a pilot project launched in Aberdeen in July 2017.

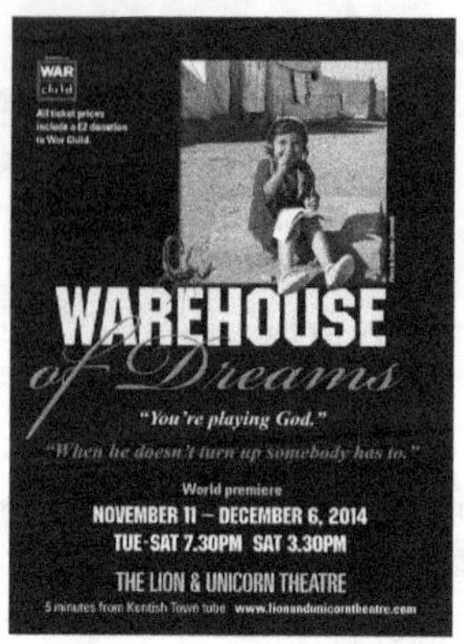

You Can't Go Home Again

I have to declare a very strong interest. My husband's play, *Warehouse of Dreams*, about the dilemmas of running a refugee camp, opens at a fringe theatre in London in November 2014. Being swept up in this event has led me to delve deeper into the topic of children damaged by war.

Every day, somewhere in the world, 30,000 people leave their homes to seek safety, and around 40% of the world's 50 million refugees are children. They have lost their home, their schooling, perhaps their family, much that has been familiar, and are now displaced within their own country or are refugees in a foreign land. They may have witnessed appalling atrocities. They see their parents disempowered. Their past is destroyed, their future is unsettled and full of threats.

Then there are the child soldiers. The courage of cabin boys on warships is lauded in poetry and prose, and the Geneva convention allows children over the age of 15 to volunteer for non-combatant roles. Many did so with enthusiasm 100 years ago when going to war appeared preferable to the misery of living in poverty at home. What seems to be a relatively recent phenomenon is the abduction of children who are then drugged and brutalised into acting as front-line soldiers or sexual slaves. Children are cheap, easy to manipulate and easy to dispose of when they have outlived their usefulness. It's estimated that over 300,000 child soldiers are being used by both rebel and government armies in more than 30 countries, and the numbers are growing.

How do you begin to build a future for millions of youngsters who have been robbed of their childhood? In 1933 Albert Einstein was instrumental in founding what is now the International

Relief Committee (IRC), one of the largest agencies working with refugees. Here in the UK, a small charity, War Child, is supporting *Warehouse of Dreams* because the play's message is about enabling children in a refugee camp to have a future.

Children arrive in camps bewildered and afraid. What they need most is a safe and stable environment. But maybe not just like home. If soldiers have burst into your living room and bayonetted your father, a place that resembles home can be very frightening. Sirens and loud bangs may evoke memories of bombs and guns. A child may have peeped through a window to see where the nice music was coming from, and witnessed an execution. Many children are numb, frozen by their fears. Some are mute. Others swing between burying their emotions and exploding uncontrollably when the pressure builds up. They need help to reduce the intensity of the memories till these lose the power to overwhelm them.

Art is a powerful tool. Many children will start by drawing experiences too horrific to put into words. Children in Dafur drew the events they had seen so accurately that their pictures were submitted to the International Criminal Court as evidence against the Janjaweed. But gradually happier images creep into their pictures and into their lives.

We all know how valuable listening to music can be when we are stressed. For young people, pop music can be a great release. Playing music, and even more creating it in a group is, as anyone who sings in a choir knows, rewarding creatively and socially, and it requires both neuromuscular relaxation and control.

Children in Za'atari, the big refugee camp in Jordan, have help from War Child. Through 15 sessions, delivered by local volunteers, using drama, games and discussion as well as art and music, they gradually settle down, open up, and learn that there are adults they can trust. They benefit from a routine. They learn to play again. They learn life skills and regain the resilience and self-confidence they will need to cope with what is inevitably an uncertain future.

Former child soldiers have all the problems of displaced children, and more. Agencies like the International Red Cross undertake to reunite them with their families, and they sometimes succeed. Locating family members is just the beginning. These children may have been forced to kill, perhaps children they grew up with or even their own families. Girls' honour has been besmirched. It takes time to persuade families to take them back.

Exchanging letters and videotapes may help to pave the way, giving confidence to the children that they can be forgiven, and to the community that the children can reintegrate. Traditional cleansing rituals are an important part of the process.

Being forgiven by their family is one thing, forgiving themselves is another. Child soldiers have to learn to live not just with what they have seen, but what they have done. It takes years. Though it's possible, even if you don't have the luck to be adopted by Emma Thompson whose former child-soldier son Tindy is now a lawyer for the UN High Commission for Refugees.

The aim for refugee children is to restart their interrupted education, and schools are a priority. But education for what? For a return home? Millions of refugee children will never go 'home'. The world's largest refugee camp is Dadaab in Kenya. There are now 10,000 Dadaab grandchildren – the children of children who were born in the camp. Organisations like War Child can equip some children for a future. The question is, how can the world give a future to 20 million refugee children?

*The video of **Warehouse of Dreams** can be viewed on www.randomthoughtslimited.co.uk*

—NASGP September 2014

Photo: Poster by Jon Anderson

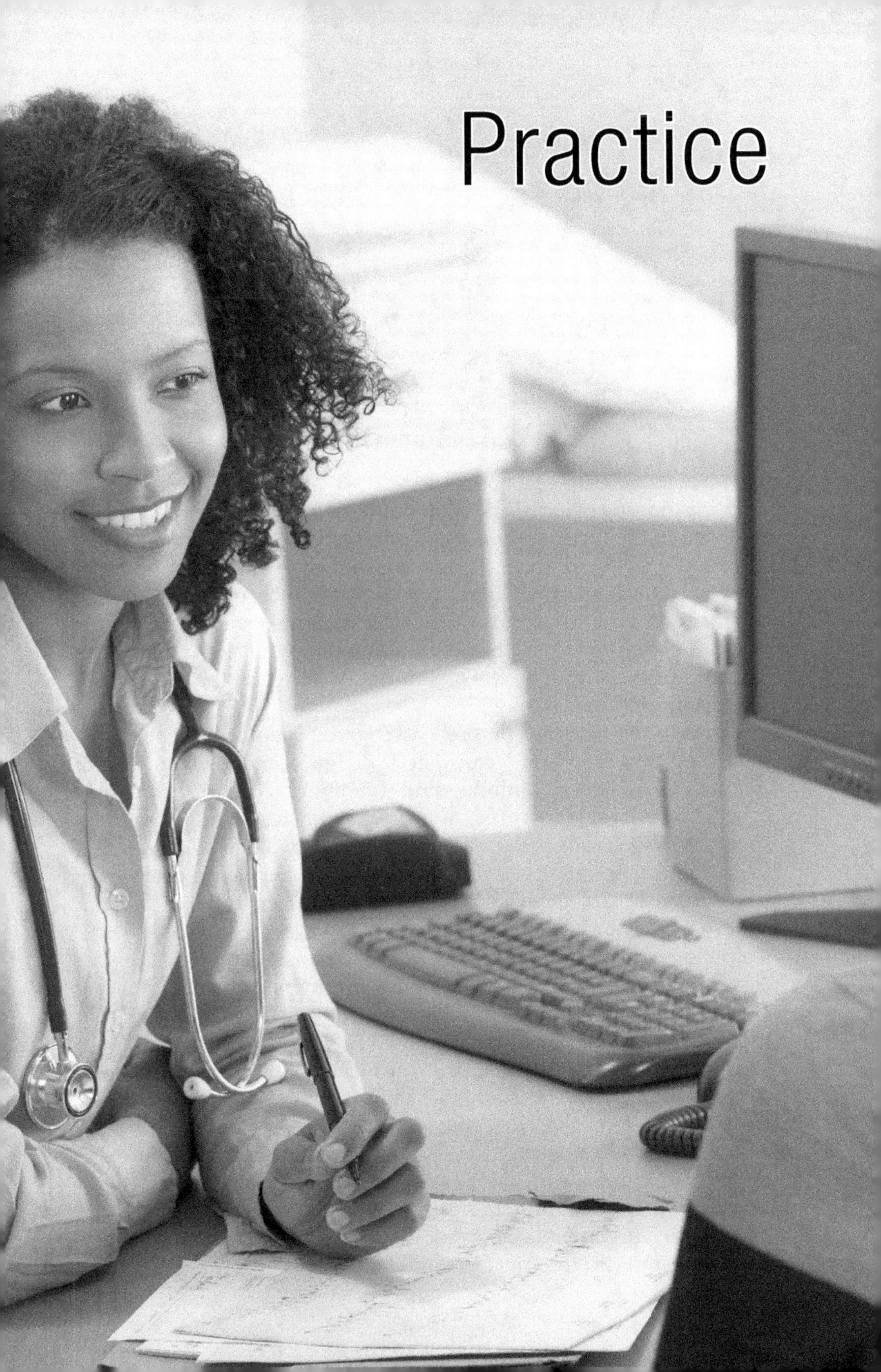
Practice

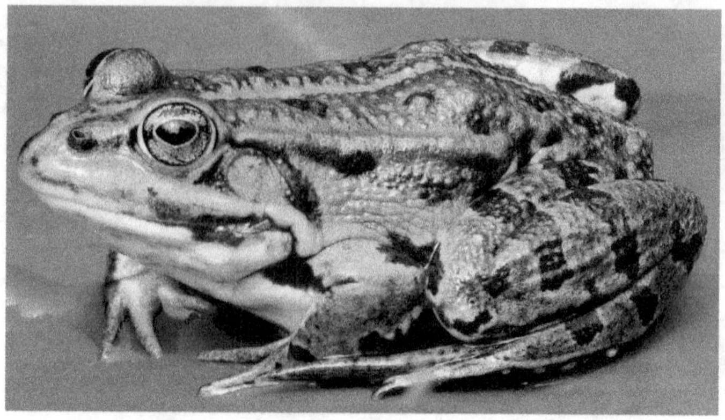

Wart-charming

At the beginning of term, a booth would be set up in the school gym. Stripped to the waist and hunched with cold and embarrassment, we stood waiting for our turn to enter the booth so that the games mistress could watch us bend forward to touch our toes. Then she inspected the soles of our feet. I don't know if she ever picked up an incipient scoliosis, but each summer verrucas condemned several girls to sitting by the swimming pool while the rest of us practised our breast stroke.

I was in my twenties before I discovered plantar warts of my own. The first crop and I co-existed for ten years. Conventional treatments achieved nothing, and toads – a traditional wart cure – were in short supply in central London. Then the warts spread to my hands. I was working in Cornwall. The nurses at the cottage hospital advised me to phone the local wart charmer. I had lived in Cornwall long enough to appreciate belief in the supernatural, and I was fed up with the warts, so I did. The telephone consultation was brief. She didn't ask many questions. A meeting was not required. My offer of payment was declined. "Leave it to me, my 'andsome", she said. I did. Within a month I was wart- and verruca-free.

I left Cornwall behind, but not the papilloma virus. A subsequent verruca resisted trial by chemicals, fire and ice. As I was walking on the edge of my foot even in shoes, I stopped telling patients that verrucas are painless. Eventually a podiatrist lasered it. Three years later, same again. Even the up-to-the-minute immune response modifier imiquimod achieved nothing. The plastic surgeon's laser generated a lot of smoke and a very large hole, but did the trick.

Last January, another one. It's on the side of my foot this time, and doesn't cause pain when walking so we are living together in a state somewhere between denial and reluctant acceptance.

Verrucas don't shorten your life, but they don't enhance your dignity, and they still worry games teachers. In the future there will be less money for the NHS. 'Efficiency savings' never seem to reduce the NHS's manifold inefficiencies, and it is services that end up being cut.

Should the NHS be treating my verrucas? A small trial – OK, my personal experience – suggests that laser excision is the most effective treatment, but the lady in Cornwall wins on cost. All other treatments scored *nul points*. But my ankle ligaments still ache after months of walking on the side of my foot. And no-one likes harbouring pests. Sometimes an attempt to help, even if unsuccessful, is valuable. So let's continue to treat verrucas.

Perhaps the Duke of Cornwall could intervene to provide wart-charming on the NHS?

—NASGP June 2009

POSTSCRIPT (2017): Two more large verrucas lasered out since 2009. Once I had fought my way through the bureaucrats' hurdles, the clinicians were very happy to help.

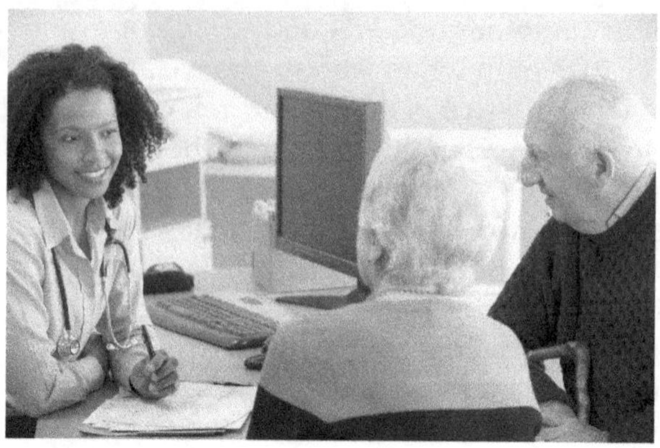

The Latest High-tech Wonder: a Checklist

Many GPs have a dim view of the intellectual gifts of surgeons. But Atul Gawande, Harvard-trained cancer surgeon, is different. He has a degree in politics, philosophy and economics from Balliol College Oxford. He broke off his medical studies to work as health adviser to Bill Clinton. During his residency he started writing for the intellectual weekly, the *New Yorker*. His two books of essays are available in the UK: *Complications: A Surgeon's Notes on an Imperfect Science* and *Better: A Surgeon's Notes on Performance*.

Of the two, I prefer *Complications*. Written during his years as a resident, it has a freshness which *Better* doesn't quite match. In *Complications*, a situation – learning to insert a central line, a case of necrotising fasciitis – triggers reflections on how we learn, how we make decisions, how we could do better. In *Better*, the established surgeon starts with a theme or a question – hospital-acquired infections, doctors and the death penalty – and subjects it to the same scrutiny. *Complications* may be more personal, but it may be *Better* with its broader scope, that can stimulate a widespread change of practice.

Managers and politicians often view medicine as an exact science and think that rigid guidelines will solve the problem of poor outcomes. "There should be no learning curve as far as patient safety is concerned", said a UK report. Gawande points out that at the front line, an imperfect science is practised by imperfect people with imperfect knowledge. We will never be right all the time, and we need to be honest with ourselves and our patients. But we can do better.

He looks hard at how. The exhilaration and mystery of getting it right, and the mundane but rewarding and often overlooked ways of improving.

There is no doubt that repeated practice and super-specialisation produce the best surgical results. Would you choose to have your hernia repaired by someone who does it day in, day out, or by a generalist, however gifted, who only repairs hernias now and again?

In some fields, the best way of achieving machine-like consistency is to use a machine. Computers beat humans at reading ECGs, for example. They aren't distracted by bleeps or over-influenced by the case they saw yesterday.

Doctors are reluctant to admit that they can be upstaged by a specialist health worker or a computer, but they should not fear that the art of medicine is thereby dead. We won't lack for emergencies where we have to rely on that sixth sense, professional intuition, for guidance, but if it fails us – fails the patient – we should have the humility to wonder how we might have done better. And humanity and kindness are as important as they ever were. Let us be glad that machines reduce the number of times we have to tell the patient, or their relatives, that we got it wrong. Let us be thankful that we are freed to concentrate on the traditional bedside role of the doctor – interpreting illness, and helping the patient make the best decisions.

Improving outcomes can be ridiculously simple in concept: standardised anaesthetic machines have reduced the risk of twiddling the knob the wrong way. But someone needs to ask the question, to collect data, to challenge the received opinion. To ask why patients at one cystic fibrosis unit in the USA did so much better than those at the other specialist centres. Could the bell-shaped curve be pushed to the right? The answer, to the amazement of those at the top of the curve was yes, it could.

Improvements can often be ridiculously cheap. But that doesn't mean they are easily adopted. Atul Gawande featured in last month's BMJ as team leader for the World Health Organisation surgical safety checklist study. The world in which we live and work is increasingly complicated. Remembering all the things you need to do when starting a prescription for the Pill is bad enough, but on ITU, where the patient's life is dependent on a hugely complex system of people and procedures, it is impossible. The WHO study found that if surgical teams used simple checklists, mistakes such as leaving sponges inside the patient dropped dramatically and lives were saved, in Toronto just as much as in Tanzania.

But why is there reluctance to adopt checklists? The NHS won't be implementing them until February 2010. Why not right away? Does the NHS need a year to save up for pencils and paper?

The truth is, behaviour is hard to change. Look at how badly hand-washing is still done: we aren't that much better than the colleagues who drove Ignaz Semmelweis from his job when he proposed that if doctors washed their hands between patients, fewer women would contract puerperal fever. Doctors' *amour propre* doesn't help. The drama of medicine is attractive – describing how you implemented a checklist isn't going to draw an awed audience in the pub – and it can be hard to admit fallibility. There is nothing in it for the pharmaceutical industry, so there is no 'free' publicity with all the inducements to change behaviour that the drug companies do so well.

What it comes down to is teamwork. We in general practice are generally better at this than many hospital teams. We are less hierarchical, more used to learning from each other. Teams in hospital tend to be less stable, but Gawande demonstrates that those who introduce themselves to each other do better than those who do not. And he suggests that however frustrating work may be, we should resist the temptation to spend coffee time moaning. It doesn't help. Instead, ask yourself a question and start collecting data . You may come up with an audit that changes practice.

📖 ***Complications: A Surgeon's Notes on an Imperfect Science***
Atul Gawande, 2002

📖 ***Better: A Surgeon's Notes on Performance*** *Atul Gawande, 2007*

—NASGP February 2009

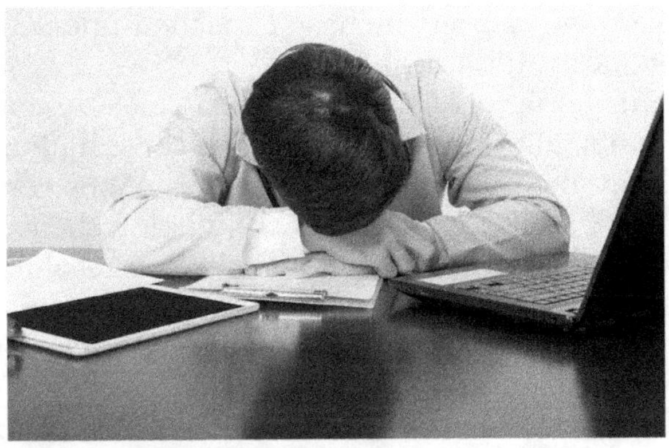

The Appointment and Exhaustion

As a student I spent two weeks in a rural GP practice. I sat in on consultations and several of the GPs asked me, in my first week of clinical training, how their colleagues handled their consultations. I realised how rarely GPs observe each other at work.

Later in my training I watched another GP make a hash of a consultation. He was abashed, but it taught me a reassuring lesson: even an acknowledged consultation expert can dig himself into a hole he can't get out of.

Since I qualified, some of the most useful tricks of the trade that I have picked up have been acquired when sitting in with other GPs. I don't mean clinical medicine, but ways of behaving, ways of putting things. But once we have finished our training, we seldom get that opportunity.

Graham Easton is a GP and a medical journalist, and he has just published *The Appointment*. He takes us through what goes on in his mind during 18 typical GP consultations. So much spins around in our head while we endeavour to present a smooth front to the patient. Graham shows the clock inexorably ticking throughout each appointment. It's a clever device; we share his anxieties about running late, and about whether he has missed something.

The consultations have been chosen to be recognisable to patients as well as GPs, and he has skillfully used them to examine issues that form the complex web of his thoughts. Our consultations are informed by our personality, our upbringing, when and where we trained, our professional and life experiences, the attitudes we have picked up, the computer's demand for QOF information and how well we slept last night. By the end of the book there are few aspects he hasn't touched upon. He displays admirable honesty. It's a page-turner.

Who is this book for? The title gives a clue: an 'appointment' is what patients talk about. GPs call them consultations. Reviews by patients say the book opened their eyes to the complexity of the job GPs do, their knowledge and skill, and the challenges of the decision-making process that leads to the resolution of each consultation. Some people in government and far too many in the press use any excuse to undermine public confidence in GPs, so I hope the publicity for *The Appointment* will boost their respect for what we do. There is a rift between science and humanity which GPs must try to bridge in every consultation, and this book shows how we can manage it.

There's a lot here for doctors, too, and for medical students. It is always fascinating to see one's own activity under the lens, especially when it demonstrates one's skills. Apart from Roger Neighbour's *The Inner Consultation*, I didn't get much out of the books on the consultation that were around when I was a registrar, but all of us, in training or old hands, will find insight and tips in *The Appointment*. It should be required reading for all students; future specialists might become rather more respectful of GPs' skills. And I wonder how many practice managers and receptionists have sat in with their GP colleagues?

One of Graham's patients says she is 'tired all the time'. Barely a day goes by without a consultation on 'TATT'. But tiredness is not just a patient's problem. Though Graham doesn't mention 'burnout', the personal cost of the job is clear. So it is interesting to consider *Exhaustion*, by Anna Katharina Schaffner. She's an academic and she examines the phenomenon of fatigue from the point of view of her field of medical humanities. I didn't find it an easy read, but here are some of the thoughts it raised.

Fatigue is often attributed to the pace of modern, technology-driven 24/7 life, a divorce from a prelapsarian existence lived in harmony with nature. But Aristotle mulled over the nature of exhaustion, and 1800 years ago some of Galen's patients may have reacted as angrily to his explanations of their problems as some of her readers have in their reviews on Amazon to Schaffner's chapter on chronic fatigue syndrome.

Every society has its TATT. But how it is named, explained and remedied depends on society, on science, on economics and on both patients' and doctors' beliefs. So it may be seen as a weakness of the muscle fibre or a defect of the moral fibre, and treated accordingly.

There's fatigue as *mal du siècle*: in the first half of the 19th century poets and artists claimed melancholia to gain their credentials as true Romantic era heroes. There's fatigue as a weapon of social control. Diagnosing Victorian women with hysteria and confining them to lengthy bed-rest may not have been a deliberate strategy for keeping them from seeking personal fulfilment, but it surely stopped them from threatening social norms.

When masturbation and homosexuality were thought to lead to fatigue (and much worse), exhaustion was a convenient threat held over people seen as social deviants. There's fatigue as a socially acceptable cover for alcoholism or for a flight from responsibility. And there's fatigue as a badge of heroism: "I'm so busy that I'm in danger of burning out".

No doubt some people complaining of fatigue have adopted the *maladie à la mode*. *Traitement à la mode* now encompasses diet, rest, exercise, medication and the relatively new kid on the block – meditation.

Exhaustion is very real and what most patients want, if they have problems that can't be identified objectively, is to be believed. Our job is to make sense of the patient's illness and find a path between collusion and conflict. More science to shed light on the biomedical aspects of fatigue syndromes would help, but until it comes along we need a lot of humanity. *The Appointment* reminds us how to play our role.

📖 *The Appointment* Graham Easton, 2016

📖 *Exhaustion* Anna K. Schaffner, 2016

—*NASGP December 2016*

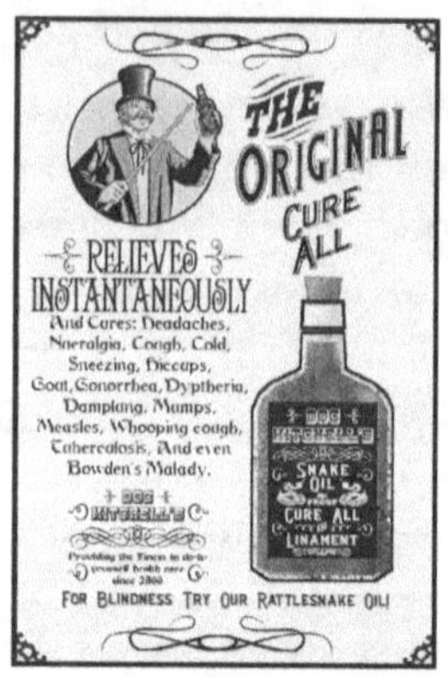

What's the Evidence for Evidence-based Medicine?

As a medical student, I attended a lecture by breast surgeon Michael Baum. At that time, how breast cancer was treated depended largely on where the patient lived and on how hard she argued for the treatment which she believed to be right. Surgeons often rejected trials because they thought they knew best; so did the patients. But I have never forgotten what Baum said: "Every woman who is not in a controlled trial is in an uncontrolled trial". Finally, his trials established what treatments work better than others, and mutilation and death rates have decreased.

As an SHO I contributed to a DRCOG revision book for junior doctors. I tried to track the origins of the words of wisdom from *Ten Teachers* that were quoted to all students and repeated in all the other textbooks. I could find no evidence to support many of the *ex cathedra* statements which determined how young doctors were going to treat their patients.

Early converts to evidence-based medicine (EBM) sometimes preached their message with an air of religiosity which irritated their colleagues. Now, when new treatments are presented we expect to see the research that supports them. So why is evidence-based medicine still so often regarded with suspicion?

Firstly, is the evidence really ALL the evidence? Dr Ben Goldacre has shown that we rarely have all the data because trials are withheld. So available data is skewed – generally in favour of the drug under consideration. His website *AllTrials* may make a difference, but meanwhile if you read a trial in which doing nothing, or providing a cheap treatment, wins over something new and expensive, believe it. Regard the rest with a raised eyebrow.

Secondly, even if all the evidence is available, how trustworthy are the conclusions? Even papers which appear to be game-changers may be re-interpreted by other statisticians, leading to very different conclusions about the appropriate clinical strategies. If you aren't a statistician, whom do you believe?

Even where analyses are based on all the available evidence and are generally supported, there are problems. If I can't understand how to interpret the statistics, few of my patients are going to. David Spiegelhalter, Professor of Public Understanding of Risk in Cambridge, knows how to get a point across. I like his nice graphics showing NNT (Number Needed to Treat) and NNH (Number Needed to Harm). Take a look at his website *Understanding Uncertainty* and play around with the animations. Find out what works for you, and so what may work for your patients.

Spiegelhalter's graphics may help you, and the patient across from you, to make decisions about treatment. But in real life how many patients are the white middle-aged male with a single problem who is recruited for trials? Mrs Hussein is 84, has at least two other chronic diseases and is already taking six different medications. Will the extra pills add to her expectation of life or to her problems? If your patient is not quite like those envisaged in the guidelines you are likely to be directed off the pathway and into a swamp of uncertainty.

Another problem with EBM is the assumption that one size fits all. David Sackett, who introduced EBM, observed that EBM is not cookbook medicine. But managers and governments like recipes. EBM provides them with yet more tools for measuring what is easy to measure about doctors' performance, not what is meaningful. EBM is about populations while GPs are treating Mrs Jones. But we are under pressure to tick boxes. So patients, whose views are supposed to be paramount, can find themselves under pressure to conform. And locums too. Do your employers ask you whether the patient was satisfied or whether you ticked the QOF boxes?

What price clinical acumen these days? Isn't that what makes an experienced doctor different from a computer? Isn't that what makes triage safer in the hands of doctors than non-doctors with algorithms? But how do you tell good judgement from dogmatic intransigence? A cynic once said that a surgeon's idea of a trial is "In my experience . . ." (one patient); "in my series . . ." (two patients); "time after time after time . . ." (three patients).

Alternative practitioners call it 'custom and practice'. When is doing something for which there is no evidence inspired and when is it like prescribing snake oil?

EBM looks backwards. Each recommendation needs to be reviewed as new evidence become available. Progress is made by challenging authority and dogma. Anecdotal medicine, good observation and making links between two hitherto apparently unconnected pieces of knowledge have to be fostered. So we need more than a register of clinical trials. We need to share and develop experience, n-of-1 trials, good ideas, speculations. We need evidence-informed medicine, in recognition that evidence-based medicine, like all tools, needs to be used with skill and judgement.

—NASGP July 2014

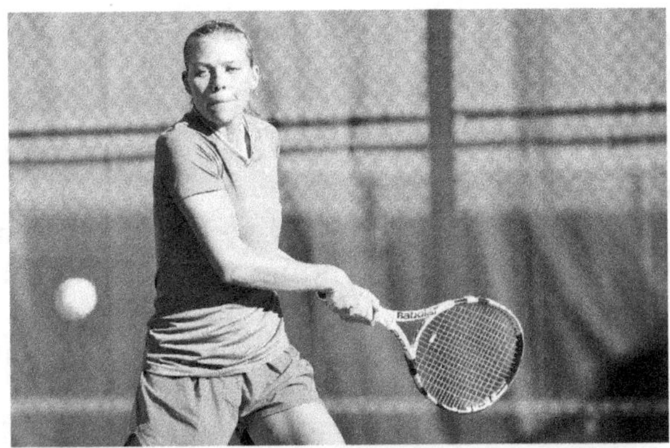

If Tennis Players Have Coaches,
Why Don't Doctors?

I make no apologies for taking a look at another article by Atul Gawande, the Boston doctor who writes common sense. In a recent edition of the *New Yorker* he asked why doctors don't have coaches.

When he turned 45 Gawande realised that his professional performance had stopped getting better. He's a surgeon, so there are obvious performance measures; he assumed he had reached his peak. Then, at a conference, he had time for a game of tennis – he's a keen player – and he took a lesson with a young coach. Gawande was amazed to find how much that one lesson improved his game. He went on to reflect that even Wimbledon champions have coaches, but surgeons don't. He wondered whether a medical coach could improve his surgery. A senior surgeon agreed to observe him operating, and suggested some simple changes in his practice, such as the way he draped the patient. Gawande's surgical performance started improving again.

Coaching, Gawande suggests, is an effective way to break entrenched habits – to teach an old dog new tricks. He quotes a study of teachers being taught new skills. After a workshop only 10% would take up a new skill. Practical demonstrations worked a little better. But when teachers had a coach watching as they tried out a new skill in the classroom, 90% of them absorbed it into their repertoire.

Students and registrars may sit in on our consultations, but as qualified GPs we are rarely observed by our peers. I recall my first two weeks of clinical training, spent in a rural GP practice sitting in with several partners. Each was incredibly curious about how the other partners consulted. They had no idea; they never saw them.

Yet there is so much to learn, both from observing and being observed. Some of the most useful 'tricks of the trade' I picked up from sitting in with other GPs, not ways of treating so much as ways of saying. For instance, how to divert patients from their long stories to possible action. Or, finding vivid ways of illustrating risk. The oil that greases the wheels of the consultation makes the difference between a mechanical exchange and a relationship. I recall one GP giving a patient test results and saying, "The results set my mind at rest; do you feel reassured?" I've used his quote for years. You don't find tips of that sort on *GPnotebook*. But how many GPs take part in a formal system for learning from each other in this way?

Recorded consultations are one way of observing. Trainers video consultations but I suspect that few of the rest of us do, and I'm not sure that it is the same as having someone in the room with you, experiencing the consultation first hand. It's too easy for someone studying a video to think they would have done better, but the observer witnessing a live consultation is sharing the consulter's dilemmas in real time. It's the difference between watching a film and a live performance.

What might you learn from trying this out? Coaches are likely to pick up some things you are already aware of, like how much time you spend looking at the computer, but may also be able to analyse when and why you turn your attention away from patients, and to suggest ways of keeping your eyes on them. And they could contribute many new insights, things you are unaware of but which make your consultation less effective. It is hard to change entrenched behaviour patterns on your own, but having a coach watch you try out new techniques does seem to help the reprogramming process.

Appraisal and mentoring can be valuable, but appraisers and mentors don't see us consulting. Maybe we could have a network of coaches – respected GPs nearing retirement or perhaps recently retired – who sit in on a surgery and talk with us about what we do well and where we could improve, whether it be the way we greet the patient, or how to consult more quickly, or improving our body language or ways of handling patients we find it hard to sympathise with. An extra bonus: they will be picking up tricks from you to pass on to others.

—NASGP December 2011

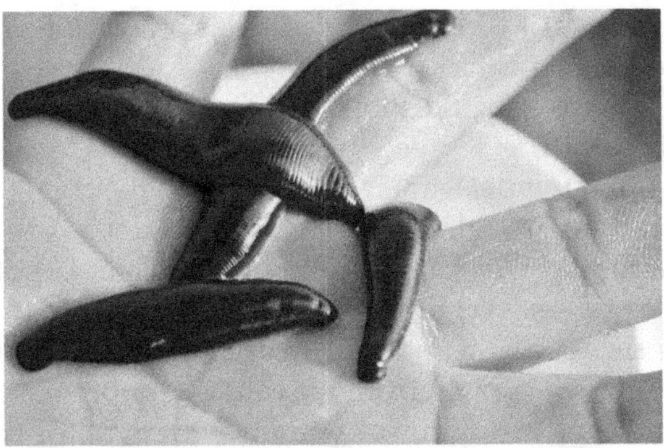

What Goes Round Comes Round

You don't need to be much over 30 to have a sense of déjà vu about the Coalition's plans to make over the NHS. I'm not going to comment on them beyond observing that it makes sense for GPs to have more say in the way services are provided, but the reality is likely to be about what services are not provided. GPs doing the rationing means post-code lottery and threatens to prejudice their relationships with patients. No doubt Andrew Lansley's vision will involve a costly upheaval, generate a few improvements, and be abandoned when the perverse incentives and unintended consequences have become apparent and another government thinks it knows better. Meanwhile, some doctors will decide to retire rather than struggle through a new set of hoops, others will hope that Britain's former colonies offer greener pastures, a few of the rest will grasp new opportunities with enthusiasm and the blessing of a government eager for backing, and most of us will sigh and carry on much as before.

Fresh oxygen reignited the embers of another smouldering health debate this week. Do statins benefit healthy people? Drug companies, which make a fortune out of statins, have been pitted against peddlers of snake oil and diets who are delighted to offer alternatives to a worried public. And cardiologists who treat patients struck down with heart disease in early middle age see things differently from GPs who know how much statins cost in patients' side effects and in their drug budgets. Evidence-based medicine ought to be a rock on which we can safely base our therapeutic decisions, but if those who are clever enough to understand the statistics can interpret the evidence so differently, what are the rest of us to think? Indeed, it appears that even highly significant results of well-conducted trials may not be reproduced if the research is repeated.

When it seems that the only certainties are death and taxes, it can be comforting to recognise that our predecessors in the profession often felt the same. Some things have changed over the years but it is remarkable how much is the same.

I came across *99 Wimpole Street* in a second-hand bookshop. The address does not exist, but former Great War surgeon J Johnston Abraham used it as the title of a series of essays published in 1937. His subjects range from novelists' ignorance of matters medical (he proposes writing a reference manual for them) to the advantages of sunlight and where to enjoy it. His reflections of the state of medical knowledge are a reminder that we too are just one frame of an unending loop.

Talking Sense is by Dr Richard Asher, former London physician – and father of red-haired actress Jane. Asher is known for describing and naming Munchhausen's syndrome, and for his insight and wit. His essays are a breath of fresh air. There is the lady who broke her leg skating on a pond and was piled with so many hot water bottles to keep her warm that she nearly sunk through the melting ice. And the ophthalmologist who suspected that a patient might have Laurence Moon Biedl syndrome and suggested referral to a physician to decide whether he had polydactyly (too many fingers).

Some beliefs have changed – we have recognised *The Dangers of Going to Bed*, for instance, though I wonder if enough attention is yet given to the effects of boredom on patients' recovery. Asher discusses *Diseases Caused by Doctors* and asks *Is Your Prescription Really Necessary?*, both topics which have grown in significance in proportion to the size of the BNF. Disease mongering was alive and well in the 1950s; we have just moved on from 'tired blood' to 'social phobia'. Use your eyes – in fact all your senses – and use your loaf, said Asher. What goes round, comes round and there are still plenty of naked emperors.

Former GP and medical writer Michael O'Donnell is in his 80s and still a rebel. *A Sceptic's Medical Dictionary* is a compendium of wit and wisdom and rapier dissection of pretension, jargon and over-valued ideas. It was published in 1997 when Mrs Thatcher's reorganisation of the NHS was grist for the mills of O'Donnell's contributors. The names may change, but human nature doesn't, and nor, it seems, do politicians' weasel words. The debunking is as current now as it was then.

So, when it all seems too much, it can help to realise that others have been through it all before. Their insight can be fortifying and their wit cheering. And remember that politicians and managers move on. Patients are always with us. Their concerns are our first priority and they don't change.

📖 ***99 Wimpole Street*** *J Johnson Abraham, 1937*

📖 ***Talking Sense*** *Richard Asher, 1972*

📖 ***A Sceptic's Medical Dictionary*** *Michael O'Donnell, 1997*

—NASGP February 2011

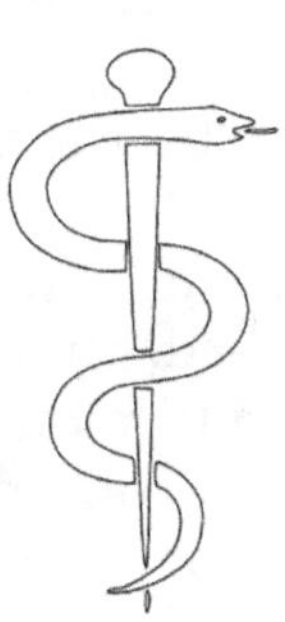

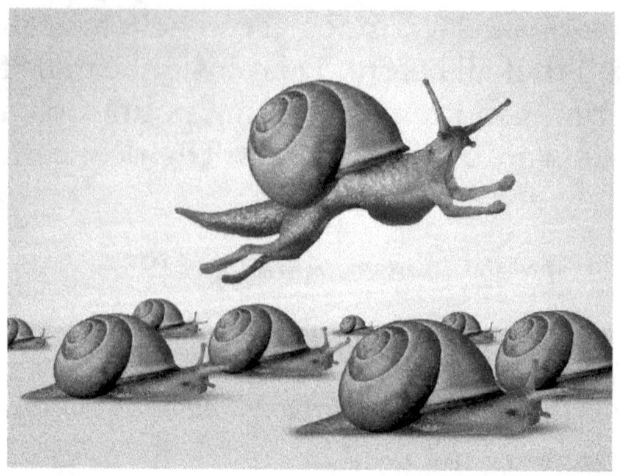

What Does It Take to Change the Game?

When is a good idea truly revolutionary? The Oxford English Dictionary defines a game-changer as 'an event, idea, or procedure that effects a significant shift in the current way of doing or thinking about something'.

If you came back to medicine after a sleep of – let's say 10 years – you'd find some crucial aspect of practice had changed in a way you would not have predicted. All your colleagues would be thinking differently. You would be obliged to learn to do things differently.

I recently wrote about self-refracting spectacles.* They were an innovative idea for patients with acuity problems in poor countries, bypassing the need for refraction by scarce optometrists before glasses can be prescribed. But they haven't caught on.

Some good ideas just don't: colour-coding asthma inhalers is common sense, but only a few countries have adopted it. Others don't fulfil their initial promise: direct thrombin inhibitors such as dagibatrin aren't yet proving sufficiently better than warfarin to change the anticoagulation game. Other innovations improve an existing game rather than changing it: surgical check lists save lives because they promote the discipline to follow established good practice. Same game, better play.

Most people would list penicillin, joint replacement, the Pill and intraocular lens replacement for cataracts as game-changers. And it was immediately obvious what a difference they would make.

But it can take time for some ideas to be adopted. In 1847 Ignaz Semmelweis proposed that deaths from puerperal fever could be reduced if doctors washed their hands between patients. But doctors resented criticism of their practice, and it wasn't until well after his death in an asylum in 1865 that his idea was accepted and maternal deaths finally fell.

Even now it can take a long time to turn the ship around. Despite sound evidence that administration of steroids to women threatened with premature labour matures the foetal lungs and greatly reduces the mortality from respiratory distress syndrome, a lot of babies died before it became standard practice.

Game-changers often mean rethinking tried and trusted ways of doing things. Clipping intracranial aneurisms used to be neurosurgeons' fun operation, but when trials of endovascular coiling were published, they recognised that embolisation by neuroradiologists is safer and more effective.

Not surprisingly some surgeons didn't reckon endoscopic surgery was here to stay. They could remove abdominal organs neatly in no time through a generous incision, and were perhaps too old to learn new tricks. But the advantages for patients, and a generation of surgeons trained in keyhole techniques, changed the game. Over the years to come, will da Vinci, the surgical robot, change operations as decisively as Leonardo changed art? If it becomes economically realistic for surgeons in Birmingham to use robots to operate on patients in Burundi, perhaps yes.

Commercial vested interests may obstruct change, and political vested interests, too. Medical use of marijuana may be a game-changer for some patients, but politicians who have campaigned on the evils of cannabis are slow to accept that idea.

There's a recent development on the funny glasses front, and it might just change that game. PEEK is an app and a cheap but clever gizmo which clips onto your smartphone and turns it into a comprehensive eye exam tool. It was developed by a British trio: an ophthalmologist, an engineer and a software geek. With PEEK on your phone you can check for cataracts, refract, and take a high resolution image of a retina. You can show the patient how the world looks to them compared with someone of normal vision. If you don't have phone reception, the information is stored till you can send the images back to ophthalmologists anywhere. Low cost, a little training, one person on a bike.

And what game-changers are on the horizon?

Gene therapy is already offering extension of life to some cancer patients but it isn't quite a game-changer – yet. 3D printing is in its infancy but seems likely to find a staggering range of applications. It's already used to create tailor-made synthetic prostheses for joint replacement and replacing bone deficits such as sections of skulls. Surgeons are using 3D modelling to plan and practise tricky operations, for example where the normal anatomy has been destroyed by tumour. 'Printing' your pills from a digital prescription, particularly useful for individualised drugs such as gene therapy, is on the horizon. The possibilities of combining with tissue engineering, scanners and 3D printing are being explored to 'print' customised heart valves, skin, intervertebral discs, kidneys – in future it may be possible to create any soft tissue organ from the patient's own cells, radically changing the transplant game.

These technologies are certainly revolutionary, even if only the wealthy will be able to upgrade all their worn body parts. True, 3D printing could permit poor countries to use recycled plastic to print small items which can be difficult to get hold of; splints perhaps. But that assumes they have the printer, the power to run it and the bits to keep it running and repair it. 3D printing technology doesn't sidestep problems of corruption and bureaucracy.

Only with the right context will a good idea translate into a game-changer. Few go viral: for better or worse change takes time.

What might change the general practice game? Small technical things, pulse oximeters for instance, change some moves in the game. And while we're waiting for 3D printing, how about an old-fashioned 2D printer that works reliably throughout a busy surgery?

Game changers don't have to be technological. What about half hour consultations? That's short by private practice standards, but would be a luxury for NHS GPs and their patients. Imagine having the time to explore the patients real concerns, to educate and explain, to consider properly with the patient how to manage the problem. More patients would leave feeling cared for, with a plan they were committed to following, and no need to return dissatisfied. Now that could really change our game.

—NASGP August 2015

* *Funny Glasses* on page 82 is about the self-refracting spectacles

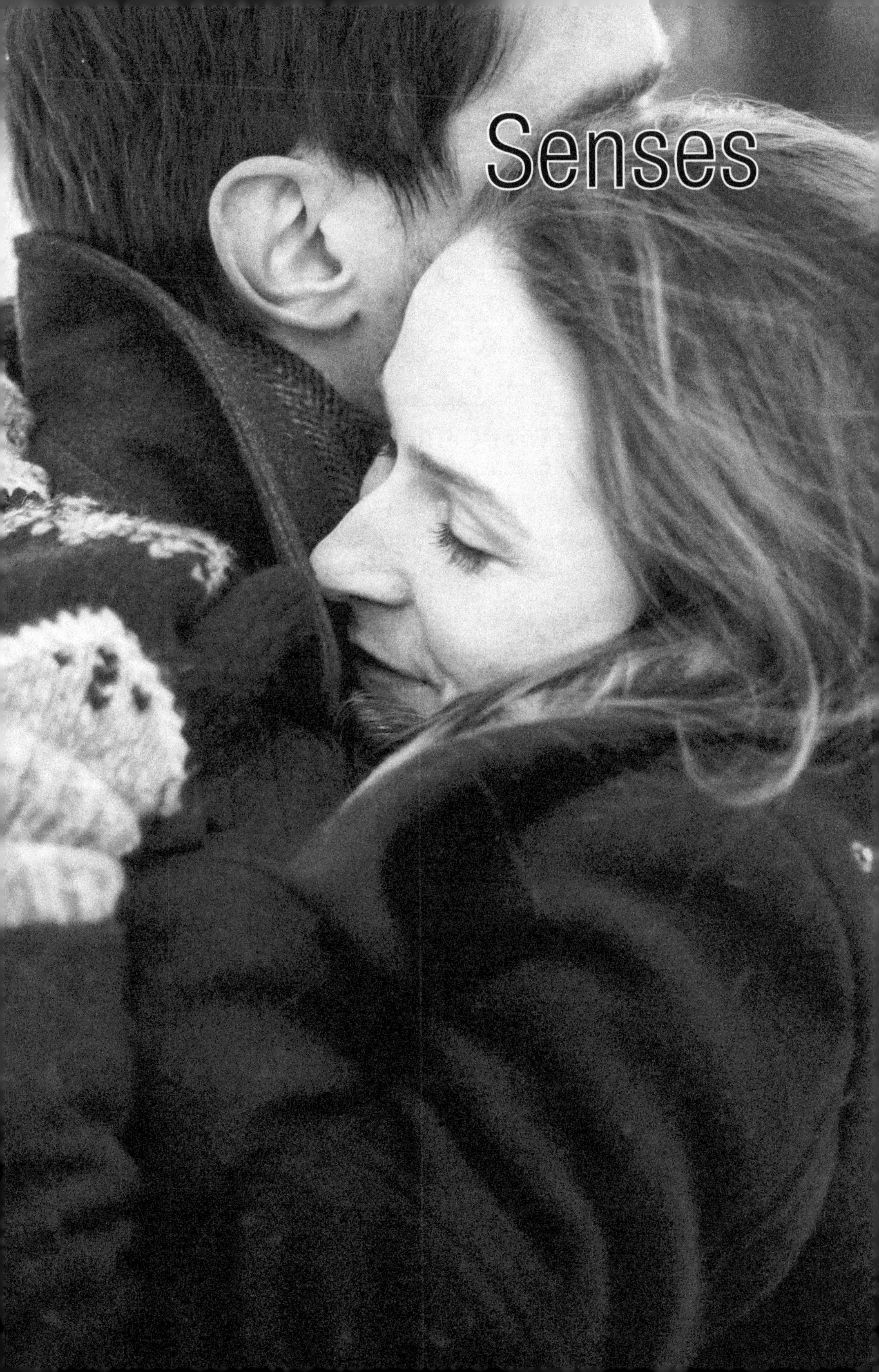

Senses

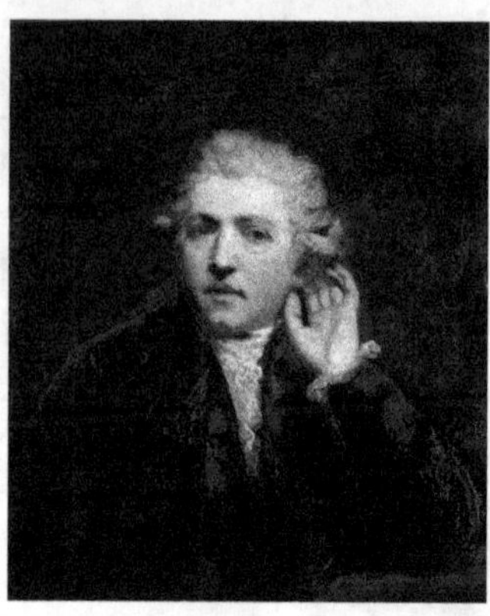

Nobody's Ever Called a *'Blind* Old Fart'

"Blindness cuts you off from things but deafness cuts you off from people." This telling insight is attributed to Helen Keller, who was both blind and deaf. Yet visual problems attract much more research money than deafness.

More than 10 million people in Britain have hearing loss. Given the ageing population and the popularity of loud music and MP3 players, it's estimated that in 20 years this figure will be 15 million.

Most of us will live long enough to know from personal experience what deafness is like: 70% of over-70s have significant hearing loss. We will enter a world of frustration. If you have lived in a country where you struggled to understand the language spoken all around you, you already know what it's like.

People have sympathy for the visually impaired. No-one is ever called a *blind* old fart. But poor hearing is equated with impaired mental and social faculties. If you don't join in you are assumed to be aloof, rude, or boring. Or demented.

Not without reason; deafness isolates people, just as dementia does. So anyone with apparent cognitive impairment should have a hearing test. An aid could be all they need to rejoin the party. And reduce their risk of developing dementia later, since untreated hearing loss is strongly associated with an increased risk of dementia. With an aid, patients who are already suffering from both dementia and deafness will be more aware, their brains more active, so they may contribute rather than confabulate.

People are unwilling to acknowledge that they have a hearing problem. "Everybody mumbles nowadays" is their excuse; it's practically pathognomonic of mild to moderate deafness. Yes, they can hear the speech, but mild high-tone deafness means they can't hear the consonants which make the words intelligible.

Nobody wants a hearing aid. People remember elderly relatives' frustrations with fiddly, whistling, ugly and unsatisfactory analogue aids. But modern digital aids can be adjusted to boost missing tones and fine-tuned for optimum effectiveness in the pub, or listening to music or for an intimate conversation. Behind-the-ear aids with an 'open ear' fitment are suitable for mild loss and avoid the problems of ear moulds. In-the-ear aids are almost invisible. There's even a fashion market for stylish coloured aids.

Too often, even state-of-the-art aids end up gathering dust in a drawer. If it's years since a patient has heard a knife dropped on the kitchen floor, they need encouragement and practice while their brain learns how to interpret the new signals.

And support must continue. An 80-year-old may check and clean her aids regularly, but by 90 she may forgetting that batteries only last a week or two and be putting her aids in the wrong ears to see if she can hear better.

Most hearing aid users will be accustomed to using the T setting on their aid to access a loop in a theatre or at a ticket window, but too few realise that loops can be fitted in homes and cars, too. And also in consulting rooms. Then there are infrared devices. They need equipment and staff trained to maintain them, but help both those with and without aids. If tour guides can use elite amplifiers – a transmitter and receiver – so can family and colleagues. Another new form of communication support is text-phoning. Apps such as NGT services (Next Generation Text) take much of the struggle out of telephone calls.

What about lip-reading? It's a chore and involves a lot of guesswork. Try saying "It is in the tin" to someone who can't hear your words and see what they make of it. It's important to clue lip-readers in to the subject you want to discuss, speaking slowly and clearly, and this is one occasion on which the lighting should illuminate the doctor, not the patient.

The NHS audiology service has a reputation, not always deserved, for being slow and providing outdated equipment. Commercial suppliers stress their no-wait services, and it is true that the NHS generally doesn't provide in-the-ear aids. But a commercial aid may cost the customer £3,000. The NHS may pay only £100 for the same model. So a well-organised NHS service with easy access is vital, and rationing hearing aids is a false economy. One RTA caused because someone couldn't hear the traffic could cost the NHS much more than hearing aids for dozens of patients.

Perhaps a third of GP consultations are with hard-of-hearing patients. As a profession we aren't good at recognising their needs. Ask yourself some questions.

- In your consultation do you ask deaf patients "How can I help you to hear?"
- How easy do you think it is for deaf patients to make appointments at the practices you work in? What could help?
- Do those practices have loops?
- Do they have an infrared system, and if so do you know how to use it?
- Can you set up a consulting room to help deaf patients hear?
- Did you know that Action on Hearing Loss (AoHL, formerly RNID) offer simple hearing tests online, or by phone on 0844-800-3838, with appropriate feedback and advice?
- Do you as a matter of course arrange a hearing test for a patient who is confused or depressed?
- What arguments do you present to a hard-of-hearing patient who is reluctant to consider a hearing aid?
- Do you know how to refer patients to lip-reading classes?
- Lip-reading classes are victims of financial cuts because they come out of the same budget as cupcake decoration classes. Could you support Action on Hearing Loss's campaign for affordable lip-reading classes in your area?
- Can you check a hearing aid and diagnose simple faults?
- Do you know what support is available for hearing aid users in your area?
- If you're looking for an audit, consider auditing a practice's deaf patients. Is their disability recorded in their notes? How satisfied are they with the service they receive? What improvements can they suggest?
- What steps are you taking to preserve your own hearing?

With thanks to Dr Ted Leverton, former GP, now an AoHL volunteer.

—NASGP February 2016

Photo: *Self-Portrait as a Deaf Man*, Sir Joshua Reynolds, c 1775, Tate Gallery

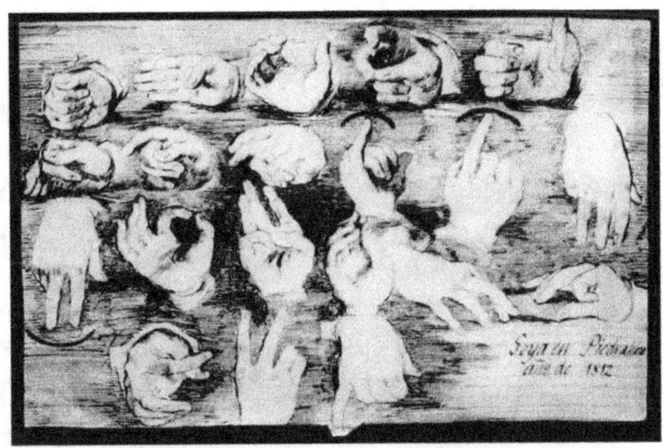

Children of a Lesser God

There are more than 800,000 people in this country who were born deaf or lost their hearing before they learned to speak. But until recently totally deaf people were obliged to struggle to talk like the rest of us. With tragic results.

It is understandable that we in the hearing world should wish the deaf to be able to join us. To communicate easily with us, and we with them, to share our aural pleasures. In 1880 an international conference passed a resolution banning the use of sign languages and proposing that deaf children should only be taught by hearing teachers. But, well-intentioned though the hearing people who drew up this 'oralist' policy were, it was a disaster for people who lacked hearing.

If you are profoundly deaf from birth you are never going to pick up a spoken language to a socially acceptable degree, any more than British retirees in Spain or old Mrs Bibi from a rural village in Bangladesh will pass as a native in their adopted country. They will always be outsiders. Deaf children were academically deprived and socially excluded, living a poor quality existence on the margins of the hearing world. In many countries they still are. Patrick, aged 15, lives in a Ugandan village. He has never had a conversation. Watch the Channel 4 *Unreported World* programme about him, and see him at his first lesson at the Deaf School, watching everyone signing. The dull expression on his face turns to joy as he realises that he too will be able to communicate.

The British Deaf and Dumb Society (now the British Deaf Society, BDA) was founded in 1886 by four Deaf men to counter the established orthodoxy and to validate the Deaf identity: deafness as a difference, not a disability. Hence the capital D. Promoting the status of signing was essential to that identity.

Signing is processed by the brain just as it processes spoken languages. There are around 150 recognised sign languages in the world, all different, so British Sign Language – BSL – and American Sign Language – ASL – have little in common. Each language has its own grammar and syntax and each develops as spoken languages do with local dialects, slang, swear words. And each, like, you know, evolves new patterns of speech, innit.

The BDA suggest that BSL is the first language for 70,000 Deaf people. That's more than speak Gaelic. For around 150,000 hearing people who live and work with Deaf people, BSL is a second or third language.

Sign language uses gesture, but it wasn't until the 1970s that it was generally appreciated that it is not miming. Only in 2003 did the British government recognise BSL as a language in its own right. Theatres, lecture halls and TV increasingly provide BSL interpreters so more of us will have had the opportunity to watch signing and to appreciate it as a fully functional language.

In September 2015, Scotland's parliament unanimously passed a bill granting BSL the protection of legal status. Westminster still has 'no appetite' to do the same. (And two years later still doesn't.)

So though Deaf people south of the border can bring their dog to a GP consultation, they still don't have the right to an interpreter. Hospitals advertise that BSL interpreters are available, but finding one is rarely as straightforward as finding someone to interpret Bengali. How easy would you find it to get hold of a BSL interpreter in the practices you work in?

Legally, deafness is a disability, but managers who would quickly be on the case if there were a problem with wheelchair access tend not to remember their obligations to the Deaf and, indeed, to the hard of hearing. Being Deaf is only the first obstacle in the way of functioning in the world of sound.

For a start, many Deaf people struggle to read and write English. It's a foreign language, and very differently constructed from BSL. Letters represent sounds, so how do you interpret words when you have no concept of a sound? Research is working on the challenge. But as with any language learning, the more fluent your first language, signing, the more easily you will learn to read English.

If you know what sounds are like, cochlear implants may make using a spoken language easier, but hearing is about more than aural input. An adult who has never heard anything will struggle to make sense of sound. So many of those who have never had hearing question the value of cochlea implants to them.

Modern IT has made communication between the Deaf and hearing people easier, but there are many Deaf people, particularly the elderly, who would find reading the newspaper or health information leaflets as difficult as I would find reading them in Greek. No wonder the Deaf have poorer-than-average health.

It surprises many hearing people that Deaf people do not crave hearing. If your English is poor, you are a second-class citizen in the hearing world. With other Deaf people they fit in. They share a rich culture. They want their children to share it. For them, deafness is normal. In another Channel 4 programme, Grayson Perry interviewed a Deaf family and their friends. Paula was brought up in Jewish culture, but to her parents' disappointment Deaf culture is now much more important to her. Deaf friends congratulate her on her Deaf daughter – "She can share your lives".

Can Deaf culture be compared with ethnic minority cultures? There is one big difference. Members of, say, the Turkish minority in UK are born to Turkish parents, but more than 90% of Deaf children are born to hearing parents. So they do not absorb Deaf culture at their mother's knee. And the Deaf cannot be distinguished by the way they dress or the food they eat.

Society's views of multiculturalism are a muddle of idealism and prejudice, fear and laziness. Can the hearing world accept the difference of the Deaf community? A 1986 Hollywood film plotted the rise and fall and resolution of a love affair between Sarah, who is Deaf, and James, who is hearing. Should the Deaf always be considered *Children of a Lesser God*?

15 and Learning to Speak *Channel 4 Unreported World, 2014*

The Deaf *Channel 4 Grayson Perry: Who are you?, 2014*

—NASGP September 2015

Photo: In middle age Spanish artist Francisco Goya suffered a severe illness which left him totally deaf. During the rest of his long life he relied on lip-reading, and, looking at portraits painted after his illness, he does appear to pay particular attention to the lips of his sitters. Did he also use sign language? Signing is recorded in 16th century Britain so equally signing may have been in use in Spain in the late 18th century. Goya's 1812 study of hands could perhaps be an illustration of a signed alphabet. But we will never know.

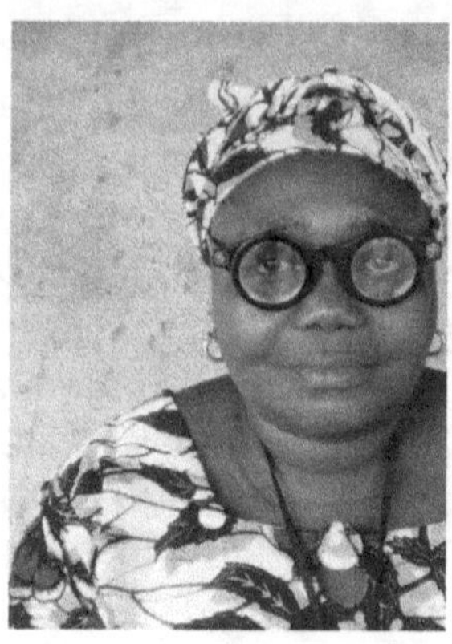

Funny Glasses

Short-sightedness isn't a disease, yet myopia is the commonest cause of poor sight worldwide. In the West, it is usually no more than a minor inconvenience alleviated by corrective eyewear, but in countries with poor infrastructure it can make the difference between a successful life and one of poverty and dependence. WHO estimates that 153 million people live with uncorrected refractive errors. The personal costs of short sight are significant. Children may be able to read a book by holding it inches from their face, but they can't read a blackboard. When they grow up they won't be able to drive. In an increasingly technological world myopia will be an increasingly serious handicap.

How can these children be provided with spectacles?

The gold standard for primary care eye services is assessment by an optometrist, who checks for eye diseases and can prescribe lenses for refractive errors. (The term optician is apparently falling out of favour and being reserved for dispensing opticians.) Every high street in the UK has several optometrists, one for every 10,000 people. Sub-Saharan Africa averages one optometrist per million people. Even relatively sophisticated South Africa, with a population of 41 million, has fewer than 300 optometrists. But refraction is only the start. Optometrists take measurements so the glasses will fit the face. Someone has to make the lenses and fit them in the frames. The spectacles have to be delivered. And they have to be affordable in countries where people on average earn only $1 a day. Refraction services are rarely free of charge. Cheap lenses are usually of poor quality. And how do you provide services and deliver spectacles in the bush?

Myopia clearly has a genetic element, and the distribution of short sight – very common in the Far East, much less common in Africa – suggests that bookwork, and these days screen-work, promote myopia. There is no hard evidence, however, and the phenomenon is not fully explained.

One vision charity estimates that 100 million children aged 12-18 in poor countries are going to need glasses if they are to get the most out of their schooling, and 60 million of them lack access to appropriate eyeglasses or to eye care professionals. Their lives will be constrained by lack of spectacles. Unless an alternative service can bridge the gap.

A possible solution is self-adjustable glasses. One version was developed by former professor of physics Josh Silver. He adapted technology used in his Oxford laboratories to produce lenses containing a membrane filled with silicone fluid. Using small syringes on the arms of the spectacles the amount of fluid in the lens, and hence its curvature, can be adjusted to the wearer's needs and then fixed by turning screws on the frame. The syringes are removed, leaving a normal-looking pair of glasses. With very little training teachers can sit pupils in front of a chart and adjust the glasses until the children can see clearly. Within minutes children have the glasses they need. It's a one-stop shop for specs for people with short or long sight. Teenagers can refract themselves. Studies in China and Boston show that self-refraction compares well with refraction by a trained optometrist.

In 2011 Professor Silver's glasses were shortlisted for the 2011 *European Inventor of the Year Award*, and won the *BMJ's* debate at the Innovation Expo conference to find the idea that would most influence healthcare in the next few years. Yet, four years later, few people have heard of self-adjusting glasses and less than 50,000 of the millions of people worldwide with acuity problems have tried them. So what are the obstacles?

Cost is a problem. Self-adjusting lenses are still more expensive than traditional lenses of similar quality. Robustness has been questioned, though current designs are said to be as able as traditional glasses to withstand the rough treatment meted out by children. Self-refraction may generate a stronger lens than is necessary, leading to headaches and eyestrain. Self-adjusting lenses come in standard frames which don't permit changing the position to fit the face and match the distance between the pupils. Acceptability is another issue. Currently, adjustable spectacles all have round frames – fine if you fancy a Harry Potter look, but not cool if everyone is wearing the same specs. In some societies, unfamiliarity with eyewear affects uptake of glasses, however provided, and children anywhere can be the butt of teasing. And even in rural Africa teenagers may judge themselves against international norms and feel that they are being offered a second-best solution; not for the rich but good enough for the poor.

Self-refraction and adjustable glasses are not the complete answer to the problem of refractive errors. They will not solve the problem of astigmatism, and without skilled assessment and fundoscopy other eye problems cannot be picked up. But in the absence of optometrists, at least short-sighted kids can get serviceable glasses and those children whose poor vision can't be corrected by spherical lenses can be identified, and then helped if services exist.

Radical ideas face big obstacles. Does this one have legs? Setting up the self-refraction one-stop shop requires organisation: education, personnel, publicity, planning sessions, training people to supervise them, arranging referral pathways for those who fail self-refraction, collecting data to assess outcomes. It's simpler than establishing a full-blown optometry service, but still requires significant investment. International agencies and governments are already committed to the optometrist model. Should they introduce an alternative service running alongside the development of conventional services, thereby diverting substantial resources from the long-term solution?

The long-term may be very long. In Malawi the first five local optometrists graduated in 2012. How long will it take this large, poor rural country to establish conventional refraction services for its 16 million people? For governments struggling to provide their people with clean water or threatened by insurgents or epidemics, what is the priority for short-sighted children?

—*NASGP April 2015*

SEE ALSO: *What Does It Take to Change the Game?* on page 72 for PEEK, a different approach to how people in poor countries can receive optometrist services.

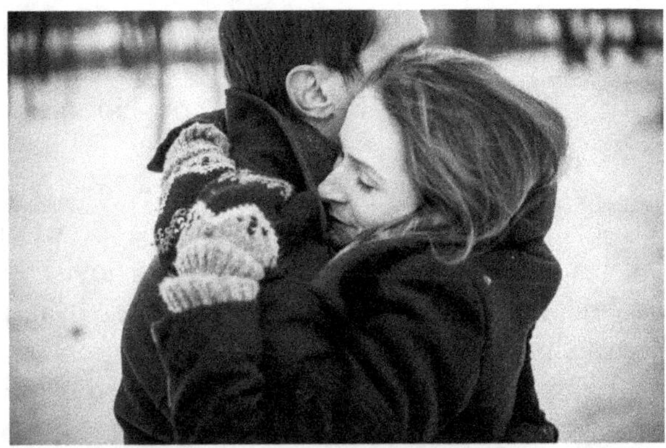

Have You Had Your Four-a-Day Today?

On YouTube Charlotte Diamond sings that *Four Hugs a Day – That's the Minimum* is what we need. And she tells us how to do it and whom to hug. Neuro-economist Paul Zac prescribes eight hugs. I don't know how either measures the effect, but there does seem to be evidence that hugs, or at least warm physical touches, benefit our mental and physical health.

Our fellow primates spend a large amount of their time on social grooming, which has been shown to be essential for group co-operation. A research study concluded that the more a basketball team high-fives, the better their performance. And we know that it is easier for people who are deaf or blind from birth to live a happy life than it is for those who lack the sense of touch. A touch, or a hug, makes all the difference when you are low, and it celebrates your highs.

Touch is the first sense that develops in utero, and we cannot grow up happy or healthy without it, but it is notably under-researched compared with other sensory modalities. The sense of touch is mediated by oxytocin through the hypothalamus so it is not surprising that touch affects the way we feel. We normally release oxytocin in response to hugs, and Paul Zac links this with the expression of empathy. The response is depressed if you are stressed, and may be absent in people who suffered abuse as children. In both of these situations normal trust and empathy are reduced or absent.

If hugs are the answer to the human condition, where do doctors stand? A BMJ search will bring up 158 entries for 'hugs'. Rule out authors named 'Hug' and you are left with a handful of personal accounts by patients, some of them doctors, of how much a hug meant at a moment of heightened emotion, or how a caring touch would have made bad news easier to bear. So we may recognise the therapeutic value of hugs, but do we consciously make use of it?

Doctors have a licence to touch patients, and doctors who touch get better ratings from patients. But we depend increasingly on technical investigations to make a diagnosis, so physical examination becomes ever more perfunctory. It isn't just the patients who may be losing out; the benefits of touch are reciprocal. As doctors' working environments become more impersonal, the more important the experience of touching a patient may be to the wellbeing of both sides.

The boundary between a professional touch and taking advantage of a patient is, well, a touchy subject. The GMC deals with many cases where doctors are felt to have overstepped the boundary, but doesn't give anything more than advice on intimate examinations. It seems that doctors, in general, wherever they trained, have similar views; refugee doctors face many cultural differences in the way medicine is practiced in Britain, but apparently touch is not one of them. So the boundary is largely set by patients. A male doctor lays a consoling hand on the arm of a female patient. In Britain today, that's sympathetic practice; in Victorian Britain, an affront; in Saudi Arabia it might be a capital offence.

Britain may appear to have embraced touchy-feely, but lots of us are hug-deficient. Many elderly people are starved of human touch. The price of self-realisation is high: in our unwillingness to make the compromises essential to living comfortably with others, families break up and people drift away from community groups. It hasn't made us happier. You can have 500 facebook friends but no-one to turn to for tea and sympathy. And a hug.

Patients' trust in doctors has been eroded by the transgressions of a small minority of our colleagues and the fall from grace of celebrities. Any touch may be misinterpreted, so we take precautions. When I trained, we rarely thought of offering a chaperone to a patient but now it's mandatory. Let's hope that it doesn't come to compulsory videoing of consultations to check for inappropriate contacts.

Dentists rarely have a problem. Since they work with assistants they have built-in chaperones, and few people get a thrill out of having their teeth filled. Sex workers, whose business is erotic touch, make a distinction between what they will do with clients and some touches – generally kissing on the mouth – are reserved for affectionate relationships.

Can anything substitute for human touch? Autistic professor of animal science Dr Temple Grandin developed a 'hug box' to give her the embraces she could not accept from human beings. Bionic arms can now give their wearers a sense of touch. The surgical robot da Vinci will soon will soon be able to feel the texture of tissues.

Maybe future generations will find e-hugs as warming as being held in someone else's arms. But till then (and I'm not sure I want to be part of that 'then') how do doctors manage the precarious balance between clinical examination and a warm human contact? With caution, of course. Explaining the nature and purpose of a clinical examination and carrying it out gently but professionally. Assessing how comfortable a patient is with closeness, their emotional state and their vulnerability.

Not all of us are huggers. But finding a warm but acceptable way of sharing a social touch is important. I always shake hands with patients when I introduce myself. It may not be the form of greeting used in the patient's culture, but it is polite in mine, and though some patients have been surprised, none has ever rejected my hand, and I feel it has got the relationship off to a good start. Others always find a reason to check a patient's pulse, a clinical examination which is not far from a handshake. But GPs can't hug everybody. So, Jeremy Hunt, how about a public health campaign for four-a-day?

—*NASGP May 2016*

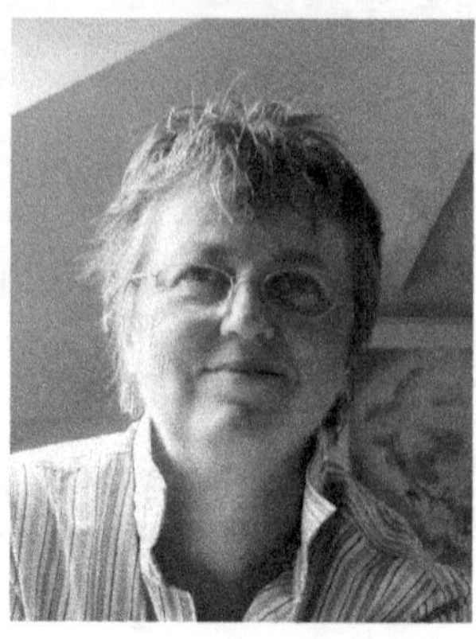

Hearing Colours

I first met Jane Mackay when she had just returned to London after two years as a volunteer teaching paramedics in Papua New Guinea. Later, when I was a mature medical student, I was able to spend a couple of weeks at her practice in Walworth, one of London's roughest areas, and her enthusiasm encouraged me to consider inner-city practice.

I knew Jane was a talented musician, but her artistic ability didn't come to public notice until she was recovering from a back injury and took up her childhood hobby of painting, because she found standing easier than sitting. Her first solo public exhibition was in Salisbury in 1993; at her Aldeburgh exhibition in 1997 I met one of the doctors from Walworth looking anxiously at the rapidly spreading rash of 'sold' spots on the pictures and muttering that she feared the practice would be advertising for a new partner before too long.

On Millennium Eve Jane removed her name from the GMC register and threw her stethoscope into the Thames. Her artistic career has blossomed. As well as her many paintings, her work now illustrates CD covers and books and has appeared as a stained-glass window.

Most of her paintings are inspired by music and determined by her synaesthesia. For her, and for the three percent of the population with synaesthesia, auditory signals are experienced both as sound and as colour. Music evokes visual images and her paintings develop them. Sometimes the images are almost unchanged in the final painting, sometimes they are the stimulus for further elaboration.

Obviously, music can evoke images for all of us, and we talk about dark base notes and light top notes. Perhaps we are all a bit synaesthetic, but for people like Jane the visual associations provoked by sounds are both consistent and particularly vivid. So Wednesday is always yellow and angular. At least it is for Jane; her sister, who is also synaesthetic, sees Wednesday as green.

Jane didn't realise that her experience was unusual, and she didn't have a name for it until the exhibition of her first big series of paintings, based on the music of Benjamin Britten, and she was talking to a psychiatrist about how the music inspired her work.

Jane's form of synaesthesia, 'coloured hearing' is the most common, but any senses can be mixed up. For a lexical-gustatory synaesthete Wednesday might always taste of corned beef and Thursday of strawberry ice cream. For other synaesthetes, elements of a series such as numbers or months are located in space, perhaps with colours attached. So Monday may be shoulder height and four feet away on the left whereas Friday is down near the right foot.

It is hard to imagine a sense that you don't have: how do you describe visual experience to the blind? So non-synaesthetes wonder what it is like and tend only to anticipate problems. Isn't there sensory overload? Apparently only rarely. Doesn't it cause confusion? No, no more than simultaneous visual and aural input confuses the rest of us. In fact, synaesthesia can give you useful extra clues. Can't be sure whether someone is from Australia or New Zealand? Instead of listening for the give-away vowels, a synaesthete may know that Australians always sound dark red whereas a Kiwi accent evokes a bright blue sensation. Maybe synaesthete doctors can use colour to help distinguish cardiac murmurs. That would have been really useful in final exams. Synaesthetes can find their gift useful when learning foreign languages. It can help with remembering vocabulary: for Jane, Friday is black-and-white check, but *vendredi* is a blue-tinged green patterned with grey. And it could be much easier to get one's tongue round pronunciation of foreign languages if strange sounds had colours attached.

For young synaesthetes, it comes as a shock to discover that other people don't know that the days of the week are coloured. In *The Chrysalids*, John Wyndham's 1955 post-holocaust novel, children with unusual sensory abilities – in the book, telepathy – are cast out of society for being mutants. Synaesthetes do not suffer that fate, but no-one I know except Jane has ever revealed themselves to be synaesthetic, and I wonder if having their experience dismissed as childhood fantasy or attention seeking deters them from talking about it, or even acknowledging it, in adult life.

Jane is not the only synaesthetic artist. It is a quality she shares with David Hockney and Wassily Kandinsky, and with musicians such as Duke Ellington and Franz Lizst. Other famous synaesthetes include writer Vladimir Nabokov and physicist (and amateur bongo drummer) Richard Feynman, for whom elements of equations had different colours.

The neurological basis of synaesthesia is not clearly understood, but functional PET scanning demonstrates that in synaesthetes with coloured hearing, but not in the rest of us, an aural stimulus excites both the aural and the visual cortices. Perhaps in most of us the synapses which link the different sensory modalities die off, or alternatively in synaesthetics the balance between neuronal excitation and inhibition is tipped towards disinhibition. So perhaps the capacity to experience a sensory stimulus in more than the conventional modality is something we are all born with. Research into synaesthesia is shedding light on brain development and organisation, and on the nature of consciousness. It may contribute to our understanding of conditions like dyslexia and autism. And maybe when we understand it better, all of us will be able to develop our potential to enjoy a multisensory experience.

—NASGP February 2007

Photo: Jane Mackay. Her website is www.soundingart.com

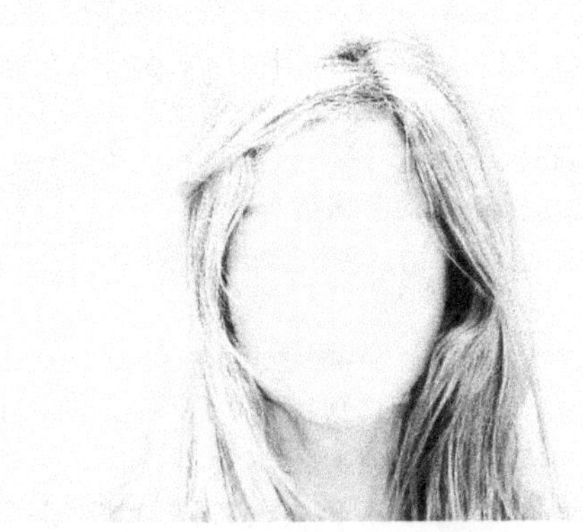

You're on the Spectrum

In the cinema, I often nudge my husband and whisper "Is this chap the same one we saw in the last scene?" and he hisses back "No, of course not!" And every time I have changed school or job, there have been a couple of people whom I continued to muddle up long after most people were as familiar to me as my family.

I'm just not very good at faces. I didn't give it any thought until 2010, when I read an article by Oliver Sacks, professor of neurology and author of *The Man Who Mistook his Wife for a Hat*. Sachs struggled to recognise anybody – patients, colleagues, friends, his family. When he discovered that a brother had the same problem, he deduced that this was probably a genetic trait.

In 1947 a German neurologist described three cases of a specific form of facial agnosia and coined the term prosopagnosia. Autopsies of sufferers showed that they all have lesions in the right visual-association cortex, but until recently face-blindness continued to be put down to shyness, absent-mindedness, bad manners, and that catch-all for any problem with interpersonal relationships, Asperger's Syndrome.

As always, for sufferers, receiving a diagnosis and knowing they are not alone make living with the condition a bit less stressful. And prosopagnosia is receiving more publicity. In 2011 consultant gastroenterologist David Fine wrote in the BMJ about the difficulties face-blindness causes him and the strategies he uses to reduce them. He manages, with some difficulty, on a day-to-day basis but networking at meetings is a near-impossible task and he feels that prosopagnosia has hampered his career. There are now blogs, discussion groups and articles in the press.

Some people can't even recognise themselves. Yet, others never forget a face. The London Metropolitan Police employs 'super-recognisers'. They scan through all that grainy CCTV footage, and from an image of a half-averted face in shadow they can recognise someone they have seen in CCTV records of crime sites, or in mug shots or even on the street five years ago. Their ability has led to the solving of 2,500 crimes last year, more than fingerprinting or DNA.

People at the extremes of a spectrum stand out. Face-blindness was described 70 years ago, but it took a while to understand that between Oliver Sachs and a super-recogniser, both two standard deviations from the mean, there is a bell-shaped curve, some people better, some worse, at recognising faces, but functioning well enough.

Take an online test to find out how good a recogniser you are. I come out as borderline prosopagnosic. I can recognise most people most of the time, under good conditions.

There are many other disease spectra. People with severe dyslexia were recognised but labelled as stupid until the condition was understood, and then it was realised that many degrees of dyslexia exist and that many people are held back by mild to moderate problems with reading and spelling, and can be helped. Autism has actually acquired the word 'spectrum' in its definition.

The recognition of spectra comes up against our wish to understand our world by classifying things.

We label people. We label ourselves: "I can't sing", "I'm useless at drawing". In reality, with the right encouragement and teaching (often sadly lacking in schools), it seems that everyone can sing or draw, not brilliantly but well enough to get pleasure out of the activity.

A lot of things are turning out to be more complicated than we used to think. Male or female? Most of us live comfortably as one or the other, but these days all sorts of states in between are recognised, not just in medicine but by law. Pregnant or not pregnant? What about the time between fertilisation and implantation? And at what point are you born? Who defines it? Religion? The law? Doctors? Is someone alive or dead? From the first time you watch a patient die you realise that dying is a process. The genotype of people with haemophilia or Downs may be clear-cut, but their phenotypes demonstrate a spectrum of consequences.

The closer you get to boundaries, the fuzzier they get. As quantum physics tells us, things are rarely black or white. Literally.

In the early 20th century, USA racial supremacists defined as 'black' anyone who was deemed to have 'one drop' of non-white blood.

If things can be defined and classified, they can be assessed and controlled. So governments need definitions.

In the old days examiners set essays, giving students the chance to roam around a topic. But essays can't be marked by computers. Multiple choice questionnaires appear to offer a range of alternatives, but I can't be the only person who has sat in an exam mutely arguing with the options.

Tick-box assessment hasn't done much to improve health care either. It is a poor proxy for judging how well GPs deal with messy reality of everyday life.

The Prime Minister is currently seeking to draw a clear distinction between people fleeing persecution – refugees, to whom we as a nation *may* show some generosity – and economic migrants – takers of advantage whom we will certainly turn away. Who is going to decide which of these desperate people should be allowed in? There is already a view that GPs should police access to the NHS. Will the government see us as assessors of right to enter the UK?

We all have a mixture of qualities and abilities at everything, positioned differently on thousands of different spectra. A complex society can't function without categories, but a humane society must recognise that life isn't black or white.

P.S. My husband points out that film directors frequently change characters' clothing and hairstyles in the middle of a film and for no obvious reason. Apparently even cameramen get confused, so no wonder viewers with prosopagnosia lose the plot! (I am delighted to note that he scored lower than I on the prosopagnosia test.)

A London University group studying prosopagnosia has an online test. You can also try Harvard's Famous Faces test.

—NASGP September 2016

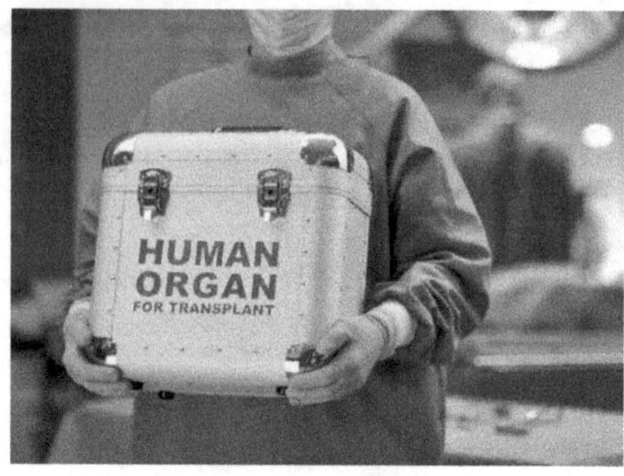

Will I Still Be Me?

Would you have a face transplant? If a dog had ripped off your nose and cheeks and lips, would you be able to learn to live with the damage, or would you consider taking on someone else's face?

Perhaps the issue that raises most anxiety is the question of identity. Psychologist Diana Sanders, waiting for a heart-lung transplant, asked "Will I still be me?" With someone else's face, how much more immediate the concern.

And it is the fear that burdens relatives of both the donor and recipient. From our face, and the way it moves, others recognise us, and even if they do not know us, they read our emotions, infer our sex, make estimates of our intellectual, social, and even moral status. After the operation, will the recipient's parents recognise their daughter? Will the donor's parents recognise *their* daughter?

It turns out that what gives our faces their recognisability is less the soft tissues than the bone structure that underlies them, so a transplant adequately matched in skin colour and texture and of the same general appearance will end up looking much more like the recipient did before the transplant than the donor. And the experience of the first face transplant recipient, in France in 2005, is that within a few months the new face gains the mobility which provides function and emotion. We 'lose face', we 'face up to things' – or not – we 'put a brave face' on something. The recipient can show her feelings; she does not feel she is wearing a mask. She might even get through passport control with her old passport. Perhaps Diana Sanders, who had lived with cardiac insufficiency all her life till she received a healthy heart, found herself more different six months after her transplant that did the French woman with a new face. "I have this huge part of someone else inside me," she said. It took her a long time to get used to the sensation of the new heart beating in her chest, to a different response to walking up stairs, to toes that were pink instead of blue.

However, there are serious downsides to face transplants. Skin is highly immunogenic and recipients of face or hand transplants need far higher doses of immunosuppression than those receiving a kidney or liver or heart. After more than 30 years' experience of transplanting internal organs it is known that 30% will develop a non-skin cancer and 80% a skin cancer, often a very aggressive squamous cell carcinoma. Premature death from cardiac problems is still common and so is chronic renal failure. The rates of these adverse effects are proportional to the dose of immunosuppressants. So if you have a face transplant you can expect to develop a severe and life-threatening chronic illness at a relatively young age.

People awaiting a liver or heart are ill and likely to die without a transplant. The most likely candidate for a face transplant is someone like the French patient: savaged by a dog, but in good general health. Is it ethical, therefore, to turn a healthy person with a damaged face into someone with more socially acceptable features but condemned to a premature death due to immunosuppression?

Would it not be better to help those who look abnormal to live a normal life? It can be done – look at Simon Weston, who was so badly burned in the Falklands. He, like many people with horrific facial injuries, became a prisoner in his own home for months afterwards. But he eventually emerged to face the world, to recognise himself and be recognised with his altered appearance, to find a new role, to be accepted by old friends and to make new ones, to marry and have children. By the time patients are being considered for a face transplant they will have been through the difficult months of horror and bereavement of their former looks and will be learning to live with their altered appearance. They will be able to face up to the face they see in the mirror. If they can't, the odds are they would not be considered psychologically robust enough for a transplant.

The problem is society's attitude to those who look abnormal. Can society alter its response to those who depart significantly from its view of what is normal, especially in these days of constant exposure to digitally enhanced role models? Maybe in former times we accommodated difference better. True, some were shunned, but many were granted special status as shamans, or at least given a protected place in the community. Could it be that we are less tolerant now, and if so is it because change is possible? A bottle of Clairol hair colour, Botox, having your Downs child's face altered surgically to make him less likely to be stared at or teased, a face transplant. Where does acceptable cosmetic improvement become morally dubious interference with nature? And whose view is it that matters?

📖 ***Will I Still Be Me?: A Journey Through a Transplant***
Diana Sanders, 2006

—NASGP June 2008

POSTSCRIPT (October 2016): Isabelle Dinoire, who received her partial face transplant in 2005, died in April 2016 after what is described as a long illness. The exact cause of her death has not been made public, but it is known that she had developed two cancers since the transplant and last year suffered an episode of rejection of the transplant which left her with only partial use of her lips. She had said that though she was determined to make the most of the opportunity the transplant had given her, she found it very difficult to adjust psychologically to having someone else's face.

Ethics

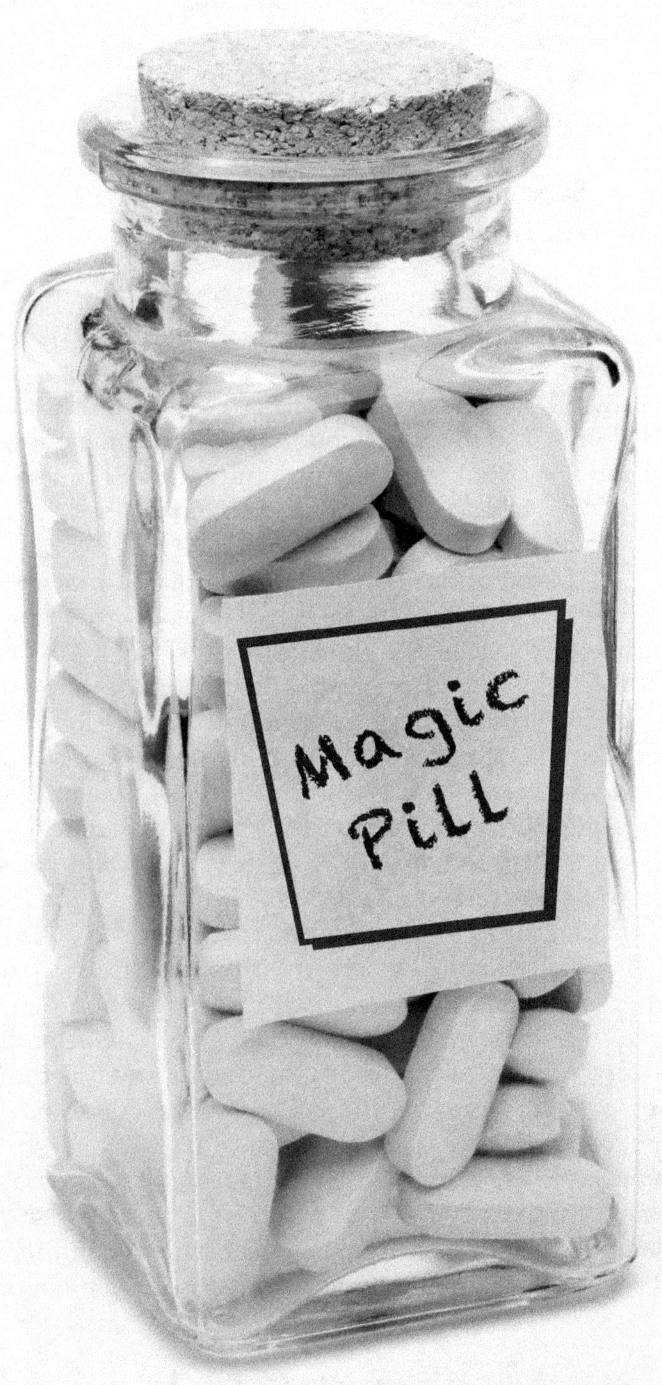

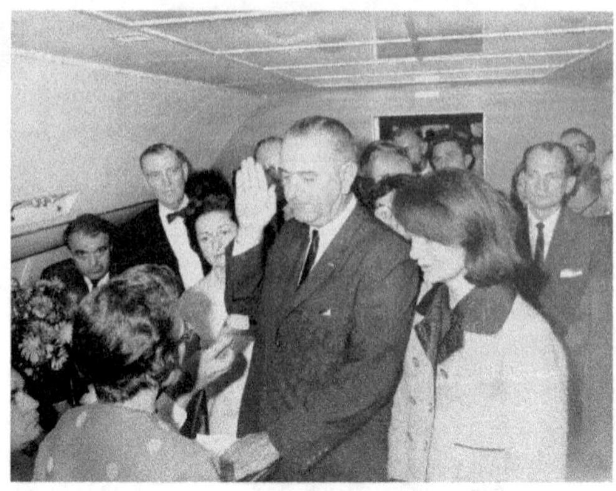

What's the Point of Swearing?

At my medical school we didn't swear an oath. Well, not a professional oath. And once I'd seen my name on the pass list, the oath I swore was never again to cross the threshold of my training hospital. The medical school didn't put on a passing out ceremony and it was left to a group of students to organise a party at which we celebrated our qualification and wished each other well in our careers.

We have all heard of the Hippocratic Oath, and many patients still believe we swear it, though they, like most doctors, have hazy and often incorrect ideas about what it says. Most US students swear a professional oath on qualification and many French students sign a written one, but apparently only about 50% of UK students are required to swear. (If it's expected of you, can you refuse, I wonder?) What is it that students are being asked to commit to, and does swearing an oath make a difference?

Professional oaths have a long history. The Hindu *vaidya's* oath dates from the 15th century BC. The Hippocratic Oath was probably written, not by Hippocrates, between the 5th and 3rd centuries BC. Oaths from Jewish philosophers, from Japan and from China, all have a long history. The Declaration of Geneva was written in 1948, after the revelations of the role of physicians in Nazi extermination camps. A recent development is the White Coat Ceremony, for students moving from the classroom to the wards for their clinical studies.

All these oaths are remarkably similar. The god they ask you to swear on may vary, but all stress that physicians' first duty is to their patients, that doctors must respect patient confidentiality, and that they must be loyal to their profession. And all oaths give some practical guidance on personal and professional conduct.

Contemporary versions of the oaths don't tamper with the statements of general principle. Putting patients first and respecting their confidentiality retain their importance. Maintaining the honour of the profession is still emphasised, even if the wording of some oaths could be interpreted as an instruction to close ranks to protect colleagues, even errant colleagues.

The most contentious sections of the oaths concern what doctors should and should not do in the course of their work. Perhaps not surprisingly. Such clauses tend to reflect the issues current at the time of writing, and so may be interpreted now as meaning something rather different from what they meant to physicians practicing in, say, ancient Greece. For instance, the traditional version of the Hippocratic Oath appears to forbid abortion. In fact, abortion was legal at that time and the oath merely advises doctors not to use unsafe methods to terminate a pregnancy. Modern oaths tend to avoid such directives, but include an ever-lengthening list of people who should not be subject to prejudice – an indication of what exercises us in the 21st century.

What is the purpose of swearing a professional oath?

When the first oaths were written, there were no registers of those considered fit to practise, so the oath was the passport to the profession. Those who had professed the oath were called professionals. People who offered medical services without having professed were quacks. Now, the rite of passage is marked by final exams, registering with the GMC and signing on with a defence organisation.

So are the oaths any more than mission statements, meaningless because no doctor would ever espouse the opposite, for instance, that patients' consultations should not be confidential? Are oaths now in fashion because there are concerns about unethical behaviour? And if so, does swearing an oath make you a more principled doctor? Surely doctors who are indiscreet with patients or who provide substandard care are not confined to the unsworn.

Still, oaths still stand for something important: the obligations that doctors feel are an essential element of their professional duty. In the 21st century we work in a managed health service where such principles are under threat. Can swearing a professional oath protect doctors from submitting to managers' demand that they put an institution's perceived needs before those of patients? Would that stand up as a defence in an industrial tribunal, a GMC hearing or the law courts?

These are unresolved questions. Meanwhile, I suggest we could revivify the oath. What if all students spent their first morning at medical school discussing the text of an oath, and then four years later, after their final exams, their last teaching session were a review of how their student experiences had changed their views? They could discuss what it means to be a professional in the 21st century. The oath would then become a living document.

Finally, the rite of passage from carefree student to responsible professional should be marked with a party to remember.

—NASGP February 2013

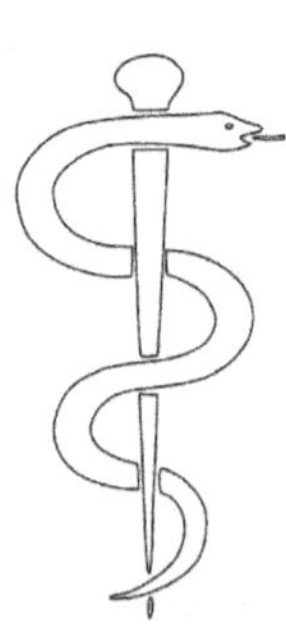

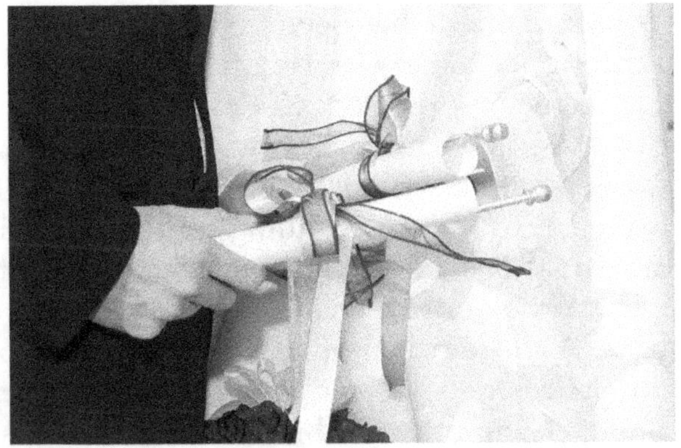

Is There Such a Thing as Informed Consent?

A patient and a doctor lying hand in hand on the operating table. That was what came to my mind as I browsed *Consent: Patients and Doctors Making Decisions Together*, the GMC's new guidance. Consent, it rightly says, is a process, and obtaining it is a partnership. But ultimately the dialogue has to come to an end, and then the patient is on his own.

A doctor who has obtained 'informed consent' has done her duty. The patient has understood the risks and benefits and thought about what they mean for him, and has made his decision. On paper, it all sounds so very rational. But real life is rarely rational. Can there be such a thing as truly informed consent?

In the bad old days, obtaining consent meant shoving a form under a patient's nose, months after their outpatient appointment and an hour before surgery. I wonder if what is now shoved is a handful of leaflets, and if so, whether they are provided in a way and at a time that actually helps the patient. Couldn't an outpatient appointment be offered after the procedure has been agreed but before surgery? That way, once the realities have sunk in patients could talk to the surgeon about their worries: the rare side effect mentioned in the leaflet, waking up vomiting after the operation, who will look after Rover while they are in hospital. Surgeons are not like timeshare salesmen, well, not usually, but a cooling off period would probably reduce the number of operations and improve the outcome of those that are performed.

Consent needs to be given with the heart as well as the brain. People smashed up in an RTA or rigid with pain from an acute abdomen just want someone to get on with the job. Where there is time for reflection, it helps if someone in the family, or a friend, or a character in a soap opera, has been through the procedure. This provides an emotional context for consent.

Consent to screening is perhaps even more fraught with pitfalls. Patients ask for a test because 'it's good to know' and 'for reassurance'. But that's not what screening is about. It is about identifying people with pathology. The trouble is the false positives. Investigations undertaken to establish that someone does not have a problem can create long-lasting damage to the body or psyche. A colleague of mine was so strongly opposed to the promotion of Prostatic-Specific Antigen tests that he vowed he would sue anyone who measured his PSA without his consent – at that time most private health screenings would automatically include PSA. That might not happen now, but the implications of screening tests are hard to comprehend, and the screening industry performs its PR well. In the USA every man is urged to know his PSA: a mildly abnormal screening test is a useful sub-total walletectomy. Doubtless, so is a total body scan, in some quarters a popular birthday gift I am told. Don't give me one.

As a GP interested in screening and its benefits and costs, I should be better placed than most to know what I might be in for. But I waved a cheery "it's nothing" to my husband when he dropped me off at the breast screening unit, and I was shaken when I was recalled. It was all right in the end, but the days before the appointment, the sitting in the waiting room, the further tests, waiting for the results, were a glimpse into hell.

Of course, it is possible to overdo the consent process. But between the choice of spending hours on pre-HIV test counselling and the 'roll up your sleeve' school of consent, there is a middle way. The challenge is to make a hypothetical situation feel real enough for the implications to sink in, and risk tables just don't do that.

When I worked for VSO, volunteers' overseas accommodation was all too often a problem. Volunteers would complain that they hadn't been warned. I would remind them of the lengthy pre-departure briefing course discussion on 'what may go wrong'. "Yes," they would say, "but you didn't tell us loud enough."

The Irish gave the Lisbon Treaty the thumbs down. It seems that the majority of the Irish support the EU, but the documents are too long, too complicated, too technical, for anyone to understand, including most of our representatives. So Eurosceptics were able to derail the approval by drawing people's attention to the bit of small print – sometimes very small – that might permit something they didn't like, be it abortion or conscription into a European army. Those emotional negatives killed off the concept of a European Union.

Marriage involves giving consent. But does being reminded barely a minute before the contract is made that the proposed union is 'for richer for poorer, in sickness and in health' count as informing of risks and giving the couple the time to reflect on their decision? Has anyone ever stopped the ceremony to ask *exactly* how big a credit card debt constitutes 'poorer'?

Context is all. Telling the world about one's health on Facebook is one thing, letting information about one's tonsillitis go on the Spine is for many people quite another.

It seems to me that useful consent is emotional consent. Sure, we need someone to run the risks past us. But we also need to feel what our decision might mean for us. That's not got much to do with 'numbers needed to treat'. It is about feelings and emotions. Perhaps a role-play should be part of the consent process?

—*NASGP August 2008*

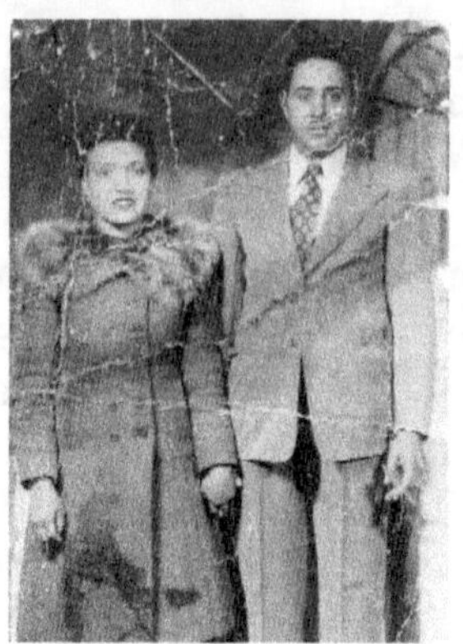

The Eternal Legacy of Henrietta Lacks

As a biochemistry student many of the experiments I studied started with a culture of HeLa cells. Why HeLa, I wondered – was it Greek?

Some years afterwards, I read that the cell line came from a patient called Helen Lane. But it turns out that wasn't her name. *The Immortal Life of Henrietta Lacks* is a fascinating portrait of a woman and her time and place, a scientific investigation, and a moral tale.

Henrietta Lacks was born in Virginia, the great-granddaughter of slaves on a tobacco plantation. Her education was cut short when she became pregnant by her cousin at the age of 14. In 1951, aged 31, with five children and syphilis, she felt a "knot" in her stomach. She went to Johns Hopkins, the only good hospital in Baltimore open to black patients. She had cervical cancer.

A tissue sample was taken before she started radium treatment. But the cells proved uniquely aggressive, both *in vivo* and *in vitro*. Even before Henrietta died nine months later, overwhelmed by metastatic cancer, the immortal cell line which bears her name was being used in labs around the world. HeLa cultures made it possible to test Salk vaccine and within a year to launch mass immunisation against polio.

Her family knew nothing of this until 1973. When they found out about the cells, they thought that in some way she was still alive. They struggled to make sense of it. The barrier between the family and the scientific community was wide, the distrust deep. It took the author of the book, an educated white woman, years to gain their trust, and to help them try to come to terms with what seemed to them yet another exploitation.

They had good reason to be suspicious. In 1932 the US Public Health Service had enrolled poor black sharecroppers from Tuskegee, Alabama in a research study, in exchange for free medical care and food. The study was the natural history of untreated syphilis. Participants were not told that, and even after the discovery of penicillin they weren't offered treatment. By the time someone blew the whistle in 1972, many had tertiary syphilis, wives had been infected and children born with hereditary syphilis, all preventable since 1947. No surprise that many black US citizens still distrust medical research and are leery of preventive medicine.

Are things different now? The Nuremberg code, drawn up in 1947 to prevent anyone using fellow human beings for experiments the way the Nazis had, didn't stop Tuskegee. And how much research is exported to poor countries where ethical codes are looser?

Henrietta's treatment was standard for 1951. Then, doctors did what doctors wanted to do and patients didn't question. As late as 1973 a postdoctoral research fellow was instructed to phone Henrietta's widower David to ask permission to take blood samples from Henrietta's relatives. The researcher – recently arrived from China – explained in poor English that they wanted to look for genetic markers. David spoke equally non-standard English. She thought he understood. He said yes because that was what you did when a doctor asked you something. The family thought they were being tested to see if they had cancer, and they waited anxiously for results which never came. The genetic marker study was published, with the family's names, but no-one thought of contacting them.

Are things different now? We know informed consent is important, but how well do we check that our patients really have understood us, and we them?

Henrietta's daughter Deborah never ceased to be troubled by the thought that her mother was still suffering somehow when her cells were blasted into space, or irradiated, or injected into prisoners, or fused with non-human cells – to Deborah 'cloning' meant making replicas of her mother.

Henrietta lived in a society where racial segregation was legal. Education, health services and prospects were limited and criminality, violence and sexual exploitation were common for those on the wrong side of the colour bar.

Are things different now? Henrietta's descendants have received no financial benefit from HeLa (and indeed cannot afford health insurance), but they are inching their way out of deprivation. And HeLa may have played a part. Traditional gospel 'soul cleansing' helped Deborah bear the burden of her mother's perceived suffering, but she realised that to understand HeLa, she needed some education. And through education Henrietta's family have come to feel proud of what HeLa has made possible – including treating the disease from which Henrietta died. Henrietta's great-granddaughter is the first Lacks to go to university.

Still, Henrietta's family remain distressed that the cells were taken and used without her knowledge.

Are things different now? It is not just in the Deep South of the 1950s that there is a gap between professionals and the public on medical ethics. Doctors at Alder Hey didn't feel that it was necessary to ask permission to remove organs at post-mortem, or even live organs if they were considered to have no value to the owner. (The thymus glands of children undergoing heart surgery were removed and sold to a pharmaceutical company.) When these practices came to light in 1999, it was clear the public felt very differently, and the result was the Human Tissue Act of 2004 and the creation of the Human Tissue Authority. Consent is now required for the use of non-anonymised human tissues for research. But the removal of Henrietta's cells would still be legal in the USA. Maybe in 50 years time, they will look askance at the cavalier way they still treat the ownership of patients' cells.

📖 ***The Immortal Life of Henrietta Lacks*** *Rebecca Skloot, 2010*

—NASGP October 2011

POSTSCRIPT: In 1972, when HeLa came to the notice of the general public, Henrietta's name was not revealed. Who was HeLa? The popular press speculated. The film star, Hedy Lamarr, perhaps? They settled on 'Helen Lane'.

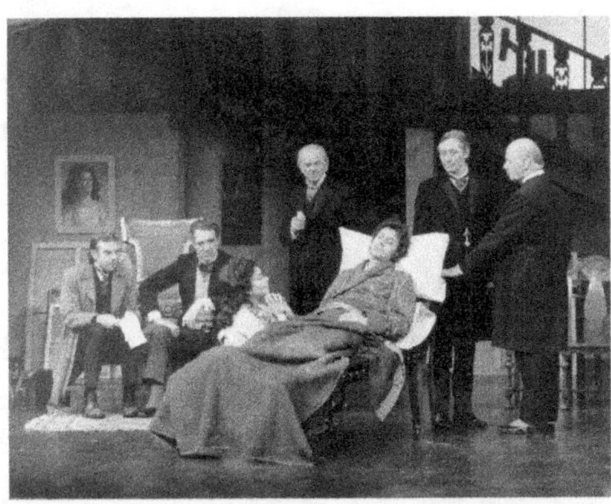

The Doctor's Dilemma – a Century Later

Bernard Shaw wrote *The Doctor's Dilemma* in 1906. What dilemma was he interested in, and how relevant is it today?

Sir Colenso Ridgeon is a distinguished doctor who has discovered a cure for TB using opsonins. He finds himself obliged to choose between treating a worthy colleague who is the one doctor in the play who looks after the poor at the expense of his wallet, and a talented but amoral artist. The artist's wife pleads for her husband and the doctor's dilemma is heightened by his realisation that he is attracted to her and would like to marry her should her husband die.

Shaw does not explore the question of professional ethics raised by the romantic attachment. Nor does he resolve the rationing dilemma, presented in terms that were highly contrived even in 1906. He uses these two personalised dramatic conflicts – *The Doctor's Dilemma* – to construct a platform for expounding his views on contemporary medical practice – all doctors' dilemmas.

The play's central message isn't really rationing. True, in many countries doctors still have to look at individual patients and choose whom to save, but someone working in a refugee camp is unlikely to feel kinship with Colenso Ridgeon. Everywhere, difficult choices still have to be made about who can be treated. In this country these have usually been taken at a managerial level, but politicians are now devolving rationing to doctors, using us as human shields when there's a row.

Shaw also introduces three of his personal hobbyhorses into the play: vegetarianism, vaccination and vivisection. But his central message is that private practice distorts healthcare and corrupts those who provide it.

First the hobbyhorses. The producers of the National Theatre's recent production have cut out most of the passing references to them. To find out Shaw's views, you have to go to the play's preface. He discusses these issues at length – well, he bangs on through 80 pages, with none of the wit of his stage play. For Shaw, a proselytising vegetarian, the eating of meat is the slippery slope to vaccination. He feels that for doctors who are seduced into thinking that vaccination is effective (or are seduced into the financial rewards of administering it) it's a small step to vivisection, and in Shaw's mind vivisection leads directly to immoral professional practice.

How relevant are Shaw's hobbyhorses today? Vegetarianism is now mainstream. Vivisection still provokes a minority to moral outrage, but animal testing, tightly controlled by law, is generally regarded, albeit sometimes reluctantly, as an essential research tool.

Vaccination against smallpox was well-established by 1906, but coverage was haphazard and there was a major outbreak in London 1901, which may have fuelled Shaw's prejudices. Immunology had made great strides in the years before the play was written, and Shaw knew about opsonins, discovered in 1903. Former students of St Mary's Hospital may recall Almroth Wright Ward, named after the doctor on whom Shaw modelled Colenso Ridgeon. Another character makes his living administering a single form immunisation – one size fits all – on the grounds that they all stimulate the immune system. Which may have been a reasonable thesis in 1906. Although Shaw's reservations are still quoted on some anti-vaccination sites, few believe that smallpox could have been eliminated were it not for vaccination, and immunisation has become a public health measure rather than a source of income for doctors.

It is how doctors' ethics are undermined by pecuniary interests that is the underlying theme of Shaw's play. His doctors are professionally arrogant. We would not see ourselves in them. *Our* practice is grounded in evidence, applied with judicious empathy. Unlike Shaw's doctors. Evidence-based medicine would have caught up with them. The surgeon in Shaw's play who makes a handsome income removing patients' nuciform sac (no, you weren't asleep in that anatomy lesson – Shaw made it up) to remove the source of blood poisoning which he believes to be the source of all illness, would soon have the GMC on his tail. Or, I hope he would. But we doctors still have our hobbyhorses, and patients are still forced into specialists' Procrustean beds. And even if doctors don't invent new diseases, drug companies certainly do.

We don't depend on selling quack treatments for *our* livelihoods. But evidence for many common treatments is still scanty. And GPs' income is increasingly tied to performance through the QOF, so part of what we do is with an eye to our income as well as our patients' interests. And it doesn't take much poking by the government to stimulate self-righteous howls from the BMA.

But we do have the NHS. So Shaw's vision of a public health service has been realised. He knew from his experience in local government just how bad was the health of ordinary people, and how little doctors and medical science contributed to improving it, and he argued strongly for a system of public health doctors. Five years after Shaw's play was premiered, the government passed the National Insurance Act which was the forerunner of today's NHS.

There is one of Shaw's wealthy doctors whose stratagem still strikes a chord. His patients are comfortably off but not rich. Compared with his colleagues his charges are modest. His dodge is to advertise 'Cure Guaranteed'. He knows he is risking trouble if the authorities notice, but they don't and, as he knows and we know, most patients will get better with time and a little support. But these days I hope we know when a patient needs the modern equivalent of opsonins.

—*NASGP October 2012*

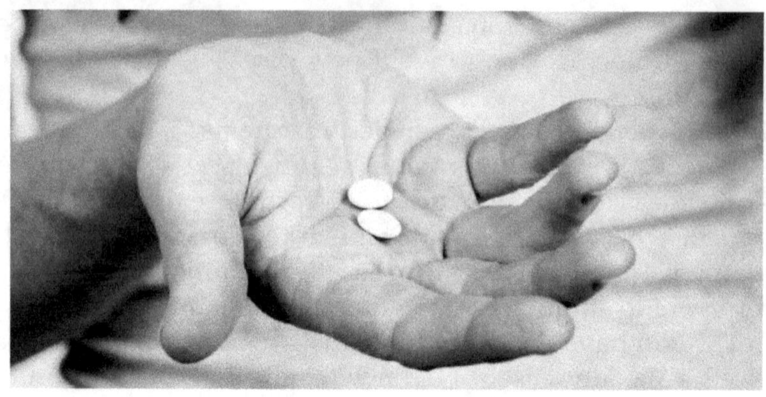

Physician, Heal Thyself?

A colleague and I were enjoying the meal before an educational event. We were registered at each others' practices, though not with each other. A viral sore throat was filling up our emergency surgeries, and we had both caught it.

"Don't tell my GP," said my colleague, "I started myself on some penicillin and I feel a lot better."

"Well, don't tell *my* GP, but *I* have been taking penicillin too, and *I* feel a lot better."

Doctors treating themselves and their families and friends is common, it's legal, and it's frowned upon.

Why do doctors self-medicate? Because they feel embarrassed admitting ill heath. Because it is easier than getting a prescription through the proper channels. Because they don't want medication on their medical record. Because they are abusing medication.

In the old days GPs rarely registered with another GP. Real GPs didn't take time off for colds, they battled on – and doubtless infected quite a few patients. Real GPs didn't suffer from depression. But some ended up sectioned or committing suicide.

In the 1990s doctors began to accept their own fallibilities. LMCs promoted the need to register with another GP, and drew up lists of GPs who would accept colleagues as patients, even if they lived out of the practice area. Now, organisations such as the Practitioner Health Programme offer doctors independent medical advice. But some self-medication still goes on. Should it be stopped?

I don't accept that self-prescribing is the slippery slope to addiction. Of all the missteps leading from upright professional to illicit opiate user, unremitting stress is a much more likely impetus than self-prescribing a course of flucloxacillin.

GPs who have self-prescribed often say they did so to save time. Self-medicating for a UTI will keep a GP in her surgery and out of someone else's. It cuts corners around an imperfectly efficient NHS. That's why I prescribed for my husband. One Sunday morning he awoke complaining of a burning pain over the ribs. O/E NAD. An hour later a band of lesions had appeared along the T10 dermatome. Shingles. We were about to leave for Argentina to trek across the Andes. I wrote him a prescription for anti-virals – he fell within the criteria so I was treating him as I would any patient – and as soon as I could I told my practice. They signed him on as a temporary resident and wished us a good holiday. Interestingly, the shingles was stopped in its tracks. Expecting the spots to go away, patients usually wait a couple of days before consulting, so it was a revelation to me how effective anti-virals can be if started early enough. I would do the same again.

Undoubtedly self-medications rarely get onto the patient's medical record. But the GMC could recommend that the prescriber inform the regular GP. And perhaps the authorities should remember that in the real world there are now a host of prescribers – hospital doctors, pharmacists, community nurses and others (let alone alternative practitioners) – and lots of their prescriptions don't get transferred into patients' medication records.

Is self-prescribing really so unethical? Ethics are slippery things. In most of Europe far more medications, including antibiotics, are available without prescription, and in much of the world you can get almost any drug over the counter. So, many doctors now practising in UK will expect to treat themselves.

The NHS devotes a lot of money to encouraging patients to self-medicate for minor problems. Surely the same applies to doctors? And doctors don't always need to write a prescription to obtain pills. How many GP migraineurs have not pocketed a drug company sample of a triptan? How many GPs have not slipped into their drawer a packet of diclofenac returned by a patient?

The GMC reminds us that putting yourself in a proper position to make a diagnosis (no car-park consultations) and knowing your limits (identifying a malignant melanoma) are essential when treating any patient. It cautions us whenever possible to avoid prescribing for family and friends. But it does not rule out prescribing even controlled drugs if they are essential to someone's medical care, urgently required and otherwise unavailable. And if you exercise proper judgement and advise the patient (including yourself) to see their own doctor if the condition doesn't respond as expected, the risks are small.

Many doctors feel that the pressure against self-prescribing is yet another case of 'nanny state'. I wonder how many builders would risk taking on a large job for family or friends. The relative expects a cut rate, but is irritated when work on his house stops because his brother-in-law has to complete a commercial contract. And if something goes wrong, it can end a relationship. So wise builders, like wise doctors, have to deal with family expectations and to recognise boundaries.

Self-prescribing is increasingly under scrutiny. A small but growing number of self-prescribing cases come before the GMC, apparently following tip-offs by pharmacists and other doctors. Predictably, benzodiazepines head the list, but antibiotics come second.

Of course, there will be occasional abuses, but making self-prescribing illegal would not prevent them. It would be another bureaucratic overreaction: responding to isolated abuses by imposing universal sanctions. We trust doctors to prescribe for other people. In an imperfect world doctors should be able to prescribe for themselves – when the circumstances justify it. Doctors make mistakes, but medical care by algorithm isn't perfect either. Doctors in general must be trusted.

—NASGP June 2012

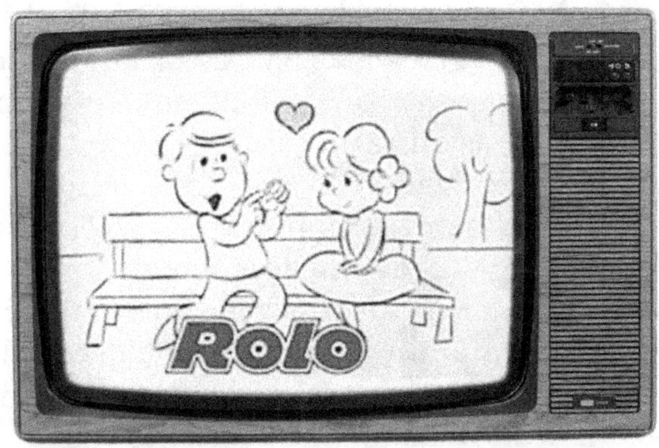

Do You Love Anyone Enough to Give Them Your Last Rolo?

A 1980s cult advertising campaign posed sharing your tube of cheap caramels as an existential crisis. A 21st-century version of the dilemma involves higher stakes. Would you offer one of your kidneys to a member of your family? To a friend? To a stranger?

The first successful living donor kidney transplant was performed in 1954. The donor and recipient were identical twins. More than half a century later, the best results come from unrelated living donors' kidneys. And end-stage renal failure is often predictable, so live donor transplants can be done before the patient needs dialysis, which improves the outcome.

No wonder that transplant units, despairing at seeing patients on the 8,000-long UK waiting list die because there aren't enough cadaver kidneys to meet the need, are keen to encourage living donation. Around 1,000 people in UK did so last year. Nearly half of renal transplants were from living donors – from spouses, blood relatives, friends, and some from unknown donors who offered a kidney to whoever needed it most.

In 2008 Annabel Ferriman, the BMJ's News Editor, described in the BMJ how she had donated a kidney to a friend. What started as a wild offer at a party ended up as a gift beyond price. Probably her experience, and the other personal stories available on donation websites, have encouraged others. Clearly, living donation is moving from a rare altruistic act, humbling to those who hear of it, towards a routine event.

The physical sequelae for the donor are said to be minor: the usual operative risks, pain which in some cases can be long term. But donors are more likely than other people to develop renal failure. In cases where the transplanted organ fails, the emotional cost for both donor and recipient can be devastating. Nevertheless the overwhelming majority of donors are very happy, even exultant, with their decision.

There is no legal obligation to donate an organ. Nor is it a requirement of any religion. And in these days of reduced social capital and fear of legal consequences, people are perhaps less likely to help a stranger in distress than they might have been when our sense of community was stronger. Nevertheless there is a growing social expectation that relatives or friends might donate a kidney. An American website urges 'End the Wait'.

In this country it is illegal to buy a kidney, and the rules make it clear that there should be no pressure on potential donors. Yet, having someone on dialysis affects the lives of all the household, and a relative or friend may be happy to donate, knowing that a transplant gives not just the patient but the whole family a better quality of life. But not everyone feels able to do so.

Potential donors may be subject to coercion. It is easy enough to weed out the businessman who brings along five employees whom he claims are willing to donate, or the patriarch who produces his teenage granddaughter. But it may be harder to detect that a young person has been encouraged to expect a generous bequest in exchange for a kidney. And it can be difficult to pick up that a potential donor actually isn't comfortable with the idea. Social pressure can be very strong. It can be seen as a test of love. Your son whose life is blighted by renal failure, or your spouse, or your father, is so hopeful. The family, the bridge club, the cronies at the pub think it is a wonderful idea. How do you get out of that?

Potential donors must be given a graceful way out, one that preserves their relationship, and the team that looks after a potential donor – which must be separate from the patient's team – should provide suitable 'alibis'.

Will living people ever become a mainstream source of spare parts? Around 2 million units of blood are donated each year. 400,000 people are on the bone marrow register. But kidneys? Donating a kidney is a much bigger deal than donating a Rolo. Are we ready to go to a dinner party and find our host eyeing us up over the risotto as a source of a replacement organ?

—*NASGP February 2010*

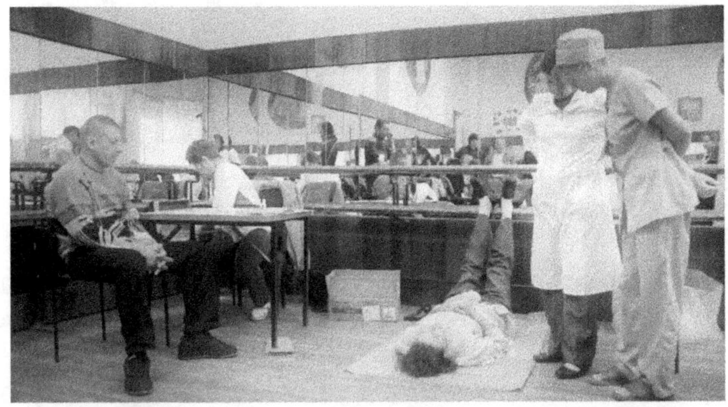

Blood Transfusion Is Safe. Isn't It?

How about a night out at the movies to watch a black-and-white documentary about a mobile blood collection unit in rural Russia? Well, *Mama Mia* it isn't, but *Blood* turned out to be fascinating.

The team cram themselves and their clobber into a beaten-up minivan and drive through wintry forests, past dilapidated wooden houses into poverty-stricken towns. They are a jolly crowd. They visit these communities several times a year and they joke with the regular donors. At supper, the vodka and the banter flow around the crowded table, and the assignations follow. Something that lost a member of the team her job. Russian authorities do not like unvarnished truth being shown on screen.

Much is familiar: dusty halls, queues of anxious donors, the occasional struggle to get into a vein, the instructions to clench the fist. There are cups of tea, too, but just for the team.

There are other differences. Donors sit upright on hard chairs. Some have just come off a night shift, others haven't the money to eat properly. Inevitably some feel faint. Their heads are shoved between their knees. It's rough and dangerous treatment, although the staff aren't unkind or, it appears, generally ill trained. It's just the way things are done.

Staff worry about meeting their 'bucket of blood' targets. They are concerned about how many units will test positive for blood-borne viruses. Potential donors are worried about being accepted. A woman without an up-to-date residency certificate is turned away. A man insists he should be allowed to donate; he's broke and he's desperate to earn the 850 rubles (£13) payment. It is clear that most donors come for the money. For some it is a lifeline. When Russia passed a law forbidding payment for donation it was repealed after five months because blood supplies dried up.

Like Russia, the USA, China and Germany pay donors. Many other countries, rich and poor, now follow WHO's recommendations that blood donation be voluntary. That's because it is safer than blood from paid donors.

Altruistic Britons provide over two million units of blood per year. They feel they are doing good, and the cup of tea and digestive biscuit may have a retro charm. Many sessions are organised at workplaces, a bit of altruism for employers, and very motivating for the team to watch the boss be the first to roll up a sleeve. Now someone is trying to make it fun: *Blood Sport* is a video game which you play while hooked up for a venesection. When you are hit, some blood is withdrawn.

There is evidence that offering payment would put off at least as many donors as it would recruit. But donors need reassurance that their blood is not sold for commercial gain. It isn't; their donations are separated into packed cells and platelets which are supplied to UK hospitals at cost price, and the NHS is self-sufficient in these products.

Nevertheless, thousands of NHS patients receive blood products from paid donors. Because of the risk of variant CJD, British plasma is not used for patients. So we import plasma products from the USA.

Thousands of plasma donations go into one dose of clotting factors or immunoglobulin. If receiving a unit of red cells is like sleeping with six people, the risk of plasma products is equivalent to sleeping with 10,000. And blood-borne infections are a growing threat. In our overcrowded global community new diseases emerge from intensive farming or make the leap from wild animals to humans, and they can spread rapidly around the world. West Nile virus, SARS, parvoviruses – what bugs are already lurking in the plasma of donors from poor countries? And rich ones?

Few countries that pay for donation maintain the high standards of screening needed for patient safely. Even if testing kits are up to standard, available, and used, turning blood into a commodity opens the door to commercial pressures. Donors are dishonest about their risk factors, companies turn a blind eye, cut corners and bribe inspectors. Plasma proteins are extracted from circulating blood by plasmapheresis. Donors can donate every few days, so it can be a regular earner. In the USA the business has a long history of scandals. If you are on Skid Row, it's a good way to pay for your next fix. China's plasma trade has an appalling record.

Blood donation has never been without risk. Early transfusions, direct from donor to patient, were fraught with problems. Later, anticoagulation using citrate reduced the risk of clotting and made possible transfusion on the First World War battlefields. Incompatibility remained a hazard, exploited in Dorothy L Sayers' 1936 short story *Blood Sacrifice*. When better cross-matching and screening became routine, the risks were all but forgotten. Then in 1983 haemophiliacs started developing AIDS.

British plasma is tainted because Mrs Thatcher's business-friendly government relaxed the safety controls on cattle-feed processing. We now import our plasma via a government-owned company. Last year, the government sold an 80% share of the business to Bain Capital, a US venture capital group. Their interests lie in making money. As with cattle feed, industry takes the profits, the public bears the risks.

This year, the Medical Research Council developed a highly sensitive blood test for variant CJD. If it proves adequate for screening donated blood we can decrease our dependency on imported plasma. But we won't be self-sufficient.

We might possibly be able to supply enough intravenous immunoglobulin (IVIG) for patients with autoimmune diseases, immunodeficiency, and severe infections. But 85% of IVIG uses are off-label. This 'wonder drug' is being tried for everything from cancer to obsessive compulsive disorder in children. Immunoglobulin from the plasma of Ebola survivors is being trialled as a treatment for Ebola. Demand around the world is rapidly outstripping supply. Desperate situations demand desperate remedies.

Monovalent autoantibodies – antibodies which target one organism – can be manufactured if the money and the will is there. But engineering IVIG products is a very long way off. The pressures on producers to exploit donors and cut corners will increase.

In myths and rituals all over the world blood has always had an ambiguous significance: giver of life and strength but always tainted with menace.

—NASGP December 2014

POSTSCRIPT: A version of this article was published in *The Guardian* on 25th January 2015 under the title *Blood money: is it wrong to pay donors?*

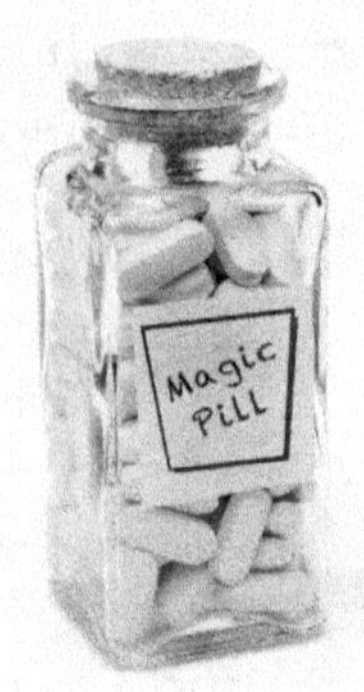

Is It Immoral *Not* to Prescribe Placebos?

Mrs Jones likes blue pills; they work better than those pink ones – even though they are the same drug. But she wouldn't touch blue mashed potato.

Wine buffs rate a wine higher if they believe it is expensive. Consumers are sure that a brand name product is superior to an identical generic, whether it be atenolol or cornflakes. The kids won't eat burned sausages at home but round a campfire they taste wonderful. Turn on a red light, and your blood pressure and heart rate will increase.

We know we are influenced by experience, by context, by sensory input, by our expectations, but most of us don't realise how open to manipulation our judgements are.

Take food. There is an art to creating expectations of food. And a science too. Oxford psychologist Charles Spence's field is gastrophysics. All our senses are involved in our appreciation of food and drink – not surprising since without them we would not survive. So Spence is investigating how our experience is shaped by our sensory input.

A £275 'ticket' (plus drinks and service) buys you 'A Journey' that a celebrity chef has contrived in a laboratory in conjunction with Professor Spence and transferred to his restaurant. There's no shortage of customers.

Spence's research also guides multinational food producers. A reassuring crunch as you open the packet makes even stale crisps taste good. Soft drinks and pre-prepared meals, and their packaging, are designed to appeal to the purchaser's senses before the product reaches their palate. And who wouldn't be glad that insights from gastrophysics about the effect of altitude and engine rumble on taste have led airlines to serve better food.

The world faces food insecurity, and overcoming cultural yuck factors could be literally vital. We all like crunchy food. Insects are an underexploited source of nutrition. It's how it's presented.

Gastrophysics has lessons for health care. After 70, our sense of smell deteriorates. Odour contributes far more to taste than our taste buds, so food needs more flavour. Increasing the contribution of the other senses can make a huge difference to how much a frail, elderly and perhaps demented person eats.

Cue mealtimes and boost the appetite by wafting the aroma of a favourite meal from a plug-in. Consider the lighting. Play sounds that have positive associations with food. Mozart for some, Meatloaf for others. Make the food more appetising by replacing soft grey glop on a white plate with coloured food or contrasting coloured crockery. Add crunch, aurally if her teeth aren't up to toast. Chat with her over her meal. And in hospitals, colour-coded trays for different diets may help staff get the right meal to the right patient, but research shows that if the tray is red, less of the food gets eaten.

There's something disturbing about how our 'objective' responses can be manipulated. It's a subject of ethical debate, and our views depend on whether we know it is happening. And on whose behaviour is being manipulated. Doctors, who aren't big consumers of fizzy drinks, generally support measures to reduce their consumption. After all, people need to be protected from themselves. The libertarian right disagrees, and orchestrates public outrage against 'nanny state'. So governments study behavioural economics and look at nudging, priming – changing subconscious cues – and other non-coercive influences on our behaviour. It has been shown that customers don't notice when the sugar or salt content of products is reduced gradually. Health by stealth works.

Some of the strategies which could arise from gastrophysics research suggest that it might be possible to massage our senses to the degree that we don't actually have to eat anything at all to feel well-fed. Already chefs produce food for Instagram rather than nutrition. Could food become a placebo?

Sounds unlikely. But we are learning a lot about placebos, and as with food our responses are summations of complex inputs to our brains. Mild hypertension and ADHD respond nearly as well to placebos as to active drugs. Sham acupuncture improves arm pain. Oxford orthopaedic surgeon Andy Carr is testing the hypothesis that many elective procedures – not just in his own discipline – are no better than placebo. Homeopaths get high ratings from patients. A study determined that two sugar pills are more effective than one.

Functional imagining shows that placebos and active drugs stimulate the same neurological pathways: Patients with Parkinson's disease given placebo treatments release more dopamine, placebo pain relievers activate the same areas of the brain as analgesic drugs and can be blocked by the same compounds. The brain areas which light up when a patient experiences side effects to real drugs are illuminated by placebos' dark cousins, nocebo effects.

All arms of a double-blind randomised controlled trial will give the participants the same care, so placebos are not just effective because the doctor is a better listener. When trials are unblinded, some patients ask to stay on the placebo. And in open-label placebo trials – where patients *know* they are receiving a placebo – patients still find that the placebo works.

A study of 252 trials of antidepressants showed an impressive NNT (Number Needed to Treat) of 1 in 3 for one drug only – placebo. Placebos won't cure cancer or heal a fracture, but given their demonstrated benefits for patients, and indirectly for doctors and the NHS, should we not be making the most of them?

Nothing destroys the doctor-patient relationship faster than deception, so patients have to know what they are getting. GPs are good at the caring aspects of the consultation, but doctors have little expertise in offering a placebo. One suggestion is "We don't know how it works but we know that some people are helped by this (sugar) pill". The same could be said of many drugs in the BNF. But we need to be confident that the evidence is firm, the GMC is supportive, the law understanding, and that a critical mass of our colleagues have learned the best way to use these powerful agents in our armamentarium.

It's an ethical conundrum. But we should accept that our neurological wiring means that total objectivity does not exist. Placebos could be more helpful and less risky than many of the expensive medications we prescribe or procedures we do.

P.S. If you fancy a whisky and have only a plastic mug to drink out of, don't broach your best single malt. It will ruin the experience. But you didn't need Professor Spence to tell you that.

📖 ***Gastrophysics: The New Science of Eating*** *Charles Spence, 2017*

—NASGP October 2017

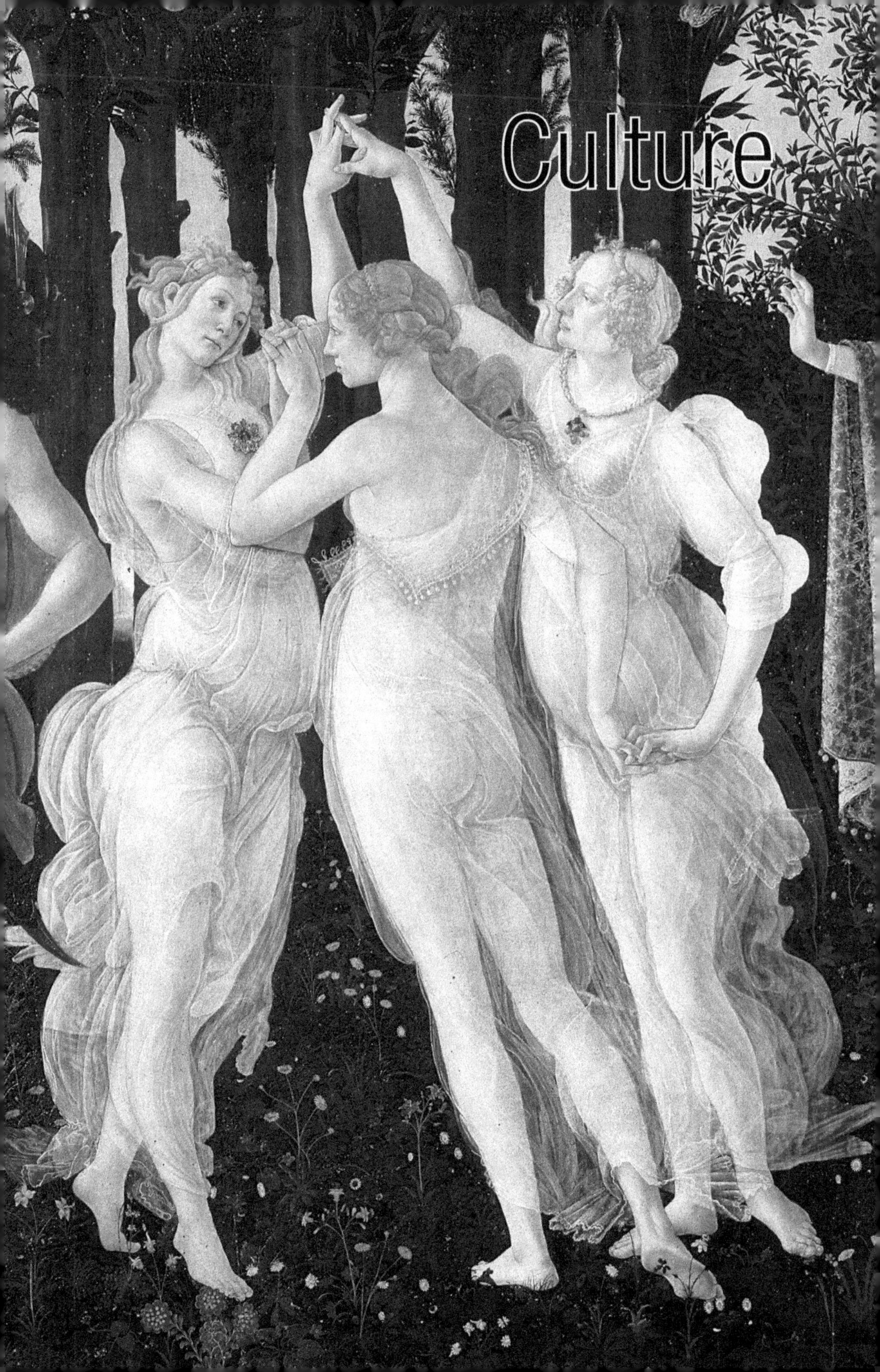
Culture

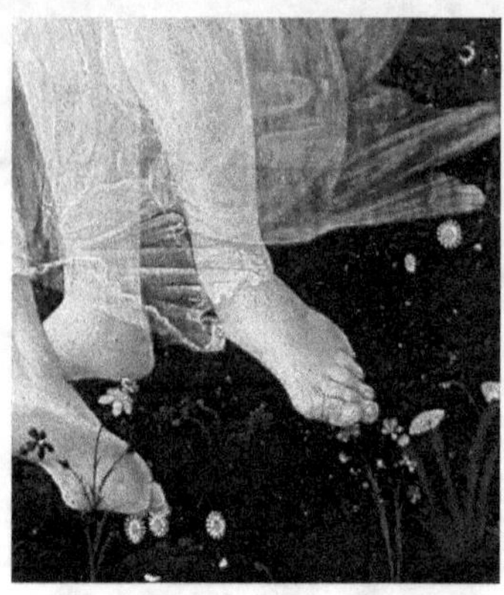

The Art of Diagnosis

Next time you're in an art gallery, see what pathology you can spot.

Diagnosis, as we know, depends on history and examination. A work of art lacks the former, but it's interesting to consider what artists notice.

In the ancient civilisations of Greece and India the sculptor's purpose was to portray human perfection. Representations of real, imperfect human beings are also rare in Egyptian art. There is a man with a withered leg, propping himself up on a staff – polio? Perhaps not coincidentally he features on a stele from the reign of the apostate pharaoh Akhenaten, who allowed himself to be depicted with a pot belly.

Religion, war and madness have long been popular subjects for European artists with an interest in disease. In medieval times, depictions of the Last Judgement reminded people that their fate in the life to come depended on their godliness in this one. The afflictions of those condemned to hell, however, owe more to the imagination of the artist than to any known pathology. But in hospitals patients saw horribly realistic images of dread diseases. The Antonine monastery at Isenheim was devoted to the care of victims of the plague and of St Anthony's fire – ergotism. Matthias Grünewald's altarpiece, painted for the monastery in 1512, shows a man rotting with sores. Christ's anguish on the cross is intensified by the pustules which cover his body. Did these portrayals of their diseases really make the sick feel less isolated in their suffering?

150 years later patients were permitted more comforting images. Murillo's painting in the Hospital de La Caridad in Seville shows St Elizabeth of Hungary carefully washing a realistically

unpleasant sore on one patient's head while another unwraps his filthy bandages.

Doctor-artists have recorded the medical consequences of war. Sir Charles Bell (he of the palsy) painted watercolours of the wounds sustained by soldiers on the battlefield of Waterloo. In the Great War, Henry Tonks, FRCS and formidable professor at the Slade School of Art, documented the work of Harold Gillies whose pioneering plastic surgery techniques restored function and a more-or-less acceptable appearance to hideously damaged faces. At the time Tonks' delicate pastels were a technical record; now they are valued as sensitive tributes both to his subjects, their appalling injuries and their courage, and to the surgeons who treated them. Julia Midgley, not a medic, has depicted the injuries of victims of 21st-century wars and their rehabilitation. She points out that, unlike a photograph, the original work of an artist 'in residence' in a war zone cannot be photoshopped for political convenience.

Madness and how societies manage it has been a popular subject. Some artworks just indulge the prurient; others bear witness to the experience of madness and to the miserable conditions of those committed to asylums. By the 20th century artists such as Edvard Munch and Frida Kahlo were portraying their own suffering, maybe somewhat self-indulgently but perhaps offering their experience to the rest of us.

Likenesses of living people begin to appear in the Renaissance and by the 17th century portraiture was a respectable way to earn a living. But artists were expected to flatter their subjects. Someone of Goya's skill might get away with being fairly honest about his king's prognathous jaw by emphasising the grandeur of his robes, but for most artists a bit of photoshopping was essential if you wanted more commissions. Hence the fame of Oliver Cromwell's demand that he be portrayed "warts and all".

Artists were more candid about themselves. Titian and Rembrandt, for example, portrayed their old age unsparingly. And they had no obligations to people who weren't paying to have their portrait painted. Look at secondary figures or imagined scenes and you can learn something about diseases of the times: club foot and other deformities that these days are surgically corrected. Rickets, perhaps. Goitre is apparently commoner in paintings by Italian artists who lived in the iodine-depleted Florentine hills than those who worked in Venice.

I recently saw a painting of a group of elderly women. Almost all had the sunken mouth of the edentulous, probably reflecting dental health at that time. But you have to be careful about making assumptions; in the 18th century rotten teeth showed that you could afford sugar.

Some artists have painted themselves in ill-health. In 2006 I wrote about Goya's Self-portrait with Dr Arrieta (see page 8). If you want to know what an elderly man in a toxic confusional state looks like, Goya's picture tells you.

Sometimes artists may record pathology without being aware of it. In Rembrandt's painting of his wife Hendrickje as Bathsheba she has puckering at five o'clock on the left breast. Breast cancer specialist Professor Michael Baum has suggested that she had breast cancer. But she continues to look healthy in later portraits until she died nine years later, apparently of plague. So maybe she had mastitis after the birth of her daughter Cornelia.

Many artists struggle to depict hands and feet. Renoir's figures so often have rheumatoid hands that it is no surprise to find that he himself suffered from rheumatoid arthritis. Perhaps he used his own hands as models and wanted to normalise them. Or, completing the details of his pictures after his sitters had gone, he may have rendered their hands in the image of his own. And look closely at *La Primavera*, above. One of the graces has hallux valgus. Whose feet was Botticelli using as a model?

Goya's portrait of the Duke of Wellington in the National Gallery was painted at the end of the Peninsula War. But unlike most portraits of victorious generals, it's not all swagger. Wellington is remote, watchful. In an earlier sketch Goya shows Wellington looking tired, pinched, withdrawn. Maybe after seven years of campaigning, he was suffering what we would now diagnose as PTSD?

Lucien Freud's portraits tend not to spare their subjects, but was he aware of the lesion on his first wife's hand – granuloma annulare, surely?

So next time you go to an art exhibition, take along your diagnostic skills, and if you identify any pathology, let me know.

—NASGP March 2016

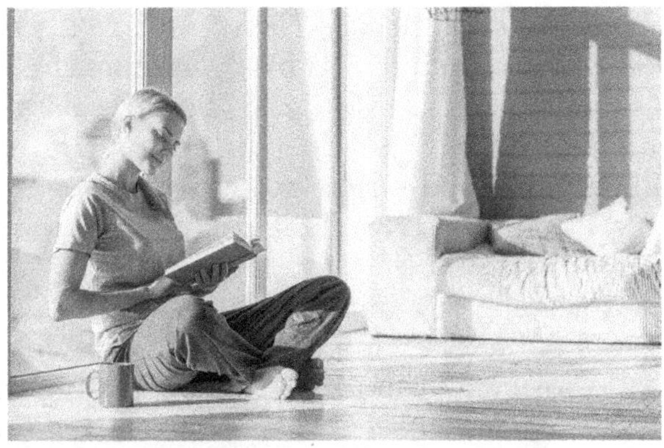

Reading for Pleasure and Profit

In 1989, Iona Heath, an inner-city GP in London, applied for study leave to spend three months reading novels. The Department of Postgraduate Education turned her down, but she took the three months off anyway and says it changed her life. The experiences of characters in fiction resonate with our own experiences, and those of our patients, and illuminate both.

There is fiction by doctors about doctors. A.J. Cronin is not currently very fashionable, but there is more to him than Dr Findley. My favourite is probably more fact than fiction: Mikhail Bulgakov's *The Country Doctor's Notebook*. While few 21st-century British doctors will experience the loneliness of making life or death clinical decisions in a remote Russian village in the middle of winter, many of us may see our own early experiences as doctors distilled in his stories.

There are doctors in fiction by non-doctors. Poor Dr Lydgate in *Middlemarch* is always quoted – ahead of his time (using a stethoscope!) but destroyed by an injudicious marriage. GPs tempted by sexual indiscretion might remember him with fellow feeling. Doctors in literature suffer other problems. Frank in Damon Galgut's Booker-nominated *The Good Doctor* or Eduardo Plarr in Graham Greene's (to my mind) much better *The Honorary Consul*, both remind us that it is not just overwork which causes burnout.

But what excited Iona Heath was not empathy with fictional colleagues. It was the human experience which novels portray. The stresses and strains of infidelity – see *Anna Karenina* in the nineteenth century or Sebastian Faulks' *On Green Dolphin Street* in the twentieth. The psychological effects of guilt – *Crime and*

Punishment and *Macbeth. La Bête Humaine*, Zola's superb study of temptation and corruption, and his even more chilling novella about guilt, *Thérèse Raquin*. Mordecai Richler's *Barney's Version* is an entertaining but telling study of the onset of Alzheimer's disease. William Horwood's *The Scallagrig* gave me more insight into what it's like to have cerebral palsy than any number of textbooks. In *The Way I Saw Her*, Rose Tremain gets into the mind of an adolescent boy, and there are times in consultations when I think of her hero Lewis and how he copes with the loss of innocence. For those who can read Spanish, I would recommend Rosa Montero's *El Corazón del Tártaro*. It is the best novel I have read this year, but not yet available in English. My Spanish is not that good but I was hooked by the suspense, the language, and the vivid picture of family dysfunction, the degradation of drug culture, and the painful path to redemption.

John Salinsky, another north London GP, sets out to tempt doctors into literature by outlining some of the pleasures awaiting those who dare to pick up the classics. He starts by analysing *A Midsummer Night's Dream*. And you didn't think it was relevant to general practice? How about conflict between children and parents (Hermia and her father), team-building (the yokel players), child custody (Titania and Oberon), the devastating effects of unrequited feelings (the lovers), the risks of eye drops when used by someone other than the patient for whom they were prescribed . . . well, that may be a lesson too far, but it is entertaining to think about what works of literature can teach us. And not just the classics. How about *Bridget Jones's Diary*?

—NASGP September 2005

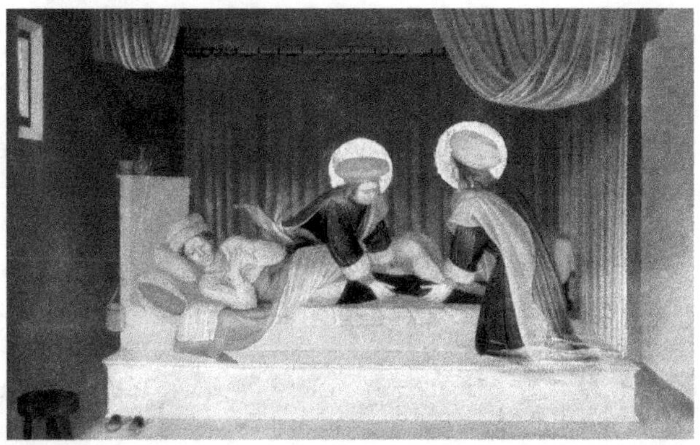

If We're Expected to Work Miracles . . .

In the small museum attached to the church in Covarrubias in northern Spain, amongst the gilded Virgins and plaster Crucifixions, I saw a strange painting. It showed a man undergoing a leg transplant. His new leg is black. Apparently the surgeons were Saints Cosme and Damian, to whom the church is dedicated. In the cathedral of nearby Burgos I saw a second painting of the same incident. And back in London I came across yet another at the Wellcome Museum.

History relates that Saints Cosme and Damian were twin doctors in third century Syria. It is said that they and their three brothers were tortured and beheaded by the Roman emperor Diocletian for their Christian beliefs. For the next few hundred years they feature in the art of both the Western and the Orthodox Church, carrying pots of ointment and triangular shoulder bags. They were termed *anargyroi* – the silverless – because they did not charge their patients.

In the Middle Ages, they start appearing as the heroes of a miracle. Justinian, a church deacon in Rome, was suffering from cancer of the leg. He dreamed that Cosme and Damian came to him and replaced his diseased leg with one from an Ethiopian Moor who had died the previous day. When Justinian awoke and saw he had a new healthy leg – although black – he knew his prayers had been answered.

In the depictions there is nothing realistic about the transplant. The brothers just slide the replacement limb into position. No blood, no instruments, only the pot of ointment. Sometimes the right leg is being transplanted, sometimes the left, apparently depending on the artistic needs of the composition. Sometimes it is an above-knee amputation, in others below-knee, and in one picture it is clear that both the severed and the new lower leg have only one bone.

In medieval times illness was seen as the punishment for sin, and only God could grant absolution and healing. The paintings were a reminder to sinful mortals that they needed the saints to speak to God for them. For two hundred years representations appear in Spain and Italy, Germany and the Low Countries, to impress the message on the congregation.

In 1517 Martin Luther pinned his protest at the sale of indulgencies to the door of the church in Wittenberg. The new Protestantism had no truck with devotion to the saints or relics. The Catholic church's response, the counter-reformation, was to clean up its act. The Council of Trent decreed that religious imagery should be restrained; art should not portray superstition. The twins and their miracle went out of fashion. In one of their few later appearances they are shown carrying out the transplant with a full set of surgical instruments and a lot of blood. But this is not simple realism. It is an advertisement: the engraving was commissioned by the Guild of Surgeons of Antwerp.

The twins' story reached Britain. A Greek Orthodox church in Camden is dedicated to them. Apparently a figure on Salisbury Cathedral carrying an ointment pot is Cosme, or is it Damian? And Damian, or is it Cosme, supports the arms of the British Dental Association. The twins remain busy today. They are said to be the patron saints of surgeons, physicians, pharmacists, dentists and day-care centres. As medics performing miracles and providing health care free at the point of delivery, should not Cosme and Damian be recruited as the patron saints of NHS GPs?

—*NASGP October 2008*

POSTSCRIPT: I keep coming across Cosme and Damian like old friends. In 2011 in Apamea in Syria I found the ruins of the first church dedicated to them. And in Crete in 2015 I picnicked under the olive trees around a tiny chapel with a carving of the twins over the door.

Photo: *The Healing of Justinian by Saint Cosmas and Saint Damian*, Fra Angelico, c 1438, Florence

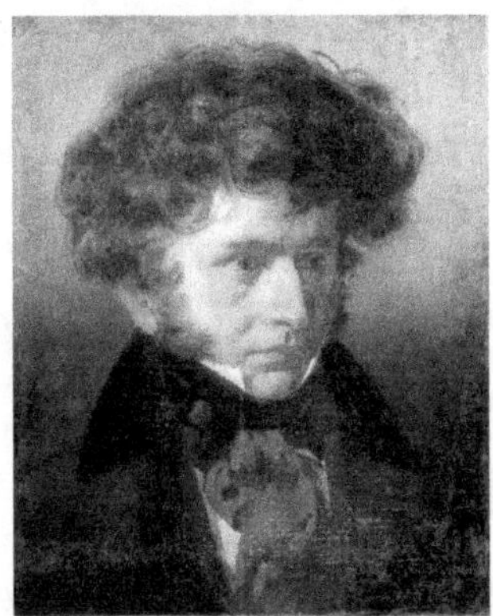

Une Carrière Fantastique

If you know anything about Hector Berlioz, it is probably that he fell in love with an Irish Shakespearean actress when he saw her playing Ophelia, and that when she spurned his advances he wrote the *Symphonie Fantastique* with its dreams of passion and nightmares of a witches' sabbath.

What is less well known is that he started training as a doctor. He came from a small town in the hills of eastern France. His father was a doctor and wanted his only son to follow in his footsteps. But young Hector – in post-revolutionary France it was still fashionable to call your children after classical heroes – knew that his future lay in music. As a boy he had found a flageolet in the back of a cupboard and learned to play it. His father was not hostile to the arts; he gave him a guitar, though he appears to have put a stop to the lessons when Hector failed his *baccalauréat*. And a new flute was the reward Hector received when, miserably, he agreed to pursue a career in medicine.

Berlioz arrived in Paris in 1821. Like many medical students, he was distracted from study by the wealth of diversions the big city offered. The orchestral concerts, and even more the spectacle of the opera, overwhelmed a passionate 18-year-old who had never before heard anything more than the band of his home town. His partner in the anatomy room tried to keep Hector's mind on study; after all they had paid for the body they were dissecting. Horrified by the smell and the rats and the sparrows squabbling over the body parts they threw over their shoulders when they had finished with them, Hector jumped out of the window. Duty to his father forced him to return, but it was to be politics that saved him. Riots closed the medical school for five months, and by the time it reopened he had signed on as a pupil of musical composition at the Conservatoire.

And that was the end of Hector Berlioz's medical career, though not the end of his conflict with his father. And it was only the beginning of a roller coaster of emotional and professional ups and downs. To enjoy such a colourful life story, you don't have to be a fan. Though you may find yourself seeking out concerts to hear the passions and frustrations pouring out in his vividly orchestrated music, and David Cairns' two-volume biography is a fantastic read.

—*NASGP January 2006*

Photo: *Portrait of Berlioz*, Emile Signol, 1832, Rome

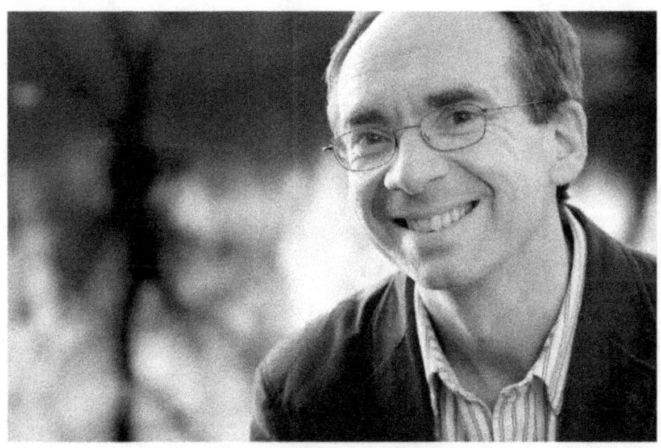

Musical Medics

Twelve years ago James Gilchrist MRCP found himself at a career crossroads: he was on a prestigious medical rotation and he had a diary full of semi-professional singing engagements. He told me how he had gone to discuss his future with his consultant. "To my surprise, this eminent physician told me he himself had always regretted not having followed his own non-medical dream. He put it to me that I might come to the end of a medical career still wondering 'What if?'" James left the rotation early to try his luck, intending to look for a new medical job if it didn't work out.

He has never returned. Well, apart from a brief test hospital locum job which demonstrated to him that while consulting, like riding a bicycle, is a skill you never lose, you need to do enough of it not to be racked with anxiety about making a mistake. He considered general practice. Sessional GPs often have several strings to their bows. "But I found I couldn't do both medicine and music properly", says James. He chose singing.

His career as a lyric tenor is assured. After a concert at the Aldeburgh Festival, a member of the audience accosted him. "I used to tell you off for humming in my operating theatre. Now I have to fork out a fortune to listen to you." But he is kept in touch with the world of medicine: his wife is a sessional GP.

Unsocial hours are less of a problem for GPs than for musicians. "Naturally, concerts tend to be held during most people's leisure time, so I am working when my sons come home from school and when they have football matches. You have to be very disciplined to book family holidays and not let an engagement, however prestigious, creep in." Continuing professional development, however, is common to both. A singer continues to take lessons, to learn both music and words, to understand exactly what those words in an unfamiliar language mean, and to work out how to perform new and strange works which make unfamiliar demands on the voice. And all self-employed people have to attend to their diary and their accounts.

Consulting is a performance art, and when you are running late with a surgery of heartsink patients, it is attractive to imagine standing before an applauding audience rather than the crowd in the waiting room, and to reflect on the different penalties contingent on missing a high C and missing a diagnosis. James's music isn't the sort that attracts the corporate hospitality crowd, more interested in schmooze than Schubert. As he looks his audience in the eyes they are wide-awake and appreciate what they hear. But however immediate and spontaneous that reaction may be, he says it isn't the same as a personal letter of thanks. "Musicians, like doctors, tend to hear from people when things go wrong, and it is wonderful when someone does write to tell me how much a concert meant to them."

James Gilchrist is one of a handful of doctors who have become full-time musicians. Alexander Borodin trained as a doctor, although he was studying the chemistry of aldehydes when he started writing music which invokes emotional reactions: listen to *In the Steppes of Central Asia*. Spending time in hospital as a child probably influenced Jeffrey Tate, born with spina bifida, to study medicine; the surgery he underwent in those years may have made possible his subsequent career as a conductor. Another conductor, Venetian-born Dr Giuseppi Sinopoli, wrote a dissertation on the connection between acoustics and the mind before turning his analytical skills to the study of musical scores. There may be other doctors hidden in orchestras, though it seems unlikely that many would give up a medical career to play second fiddle.

Music may be less obviously useful than medicine, but it has an important place in most people's lives. *Desert Island Discs* hasn't been going for 67 years for nothing. And the effects of music can be profound: I was in a sultry Royal Albert Hall the day the Soviet tanks crushed the Prague Spring. The USSR State Orchestra was about to play the cello concerto by Antonín Dvořák. A Czech. The atmosphere in the hall, like the weather outside, was electric. There were taunts from the audience. Then someone shouted "Let them play". And they did. With what passion. The soloist, Mtsislav Rostropovich, seemed to be in tears as he played, uniting the audience and the orchestra in an emotional experience of shared humanity. Later, Rostropovich defected to the West.

Music can reach us when we are beyond the comfort of words. Music therapy has proved a valuable help to people suffering from almost any health problem, most obviously psychiatric disorders, neurological disease, development disability, and of course stress, but also medical problems. James Gilchrist calls music the medicine of the soul.

—NASGP April 2009

POSTSCRIPT: Sir Jeffrey Tate died in August 2017.

Photo: James Gilchrist

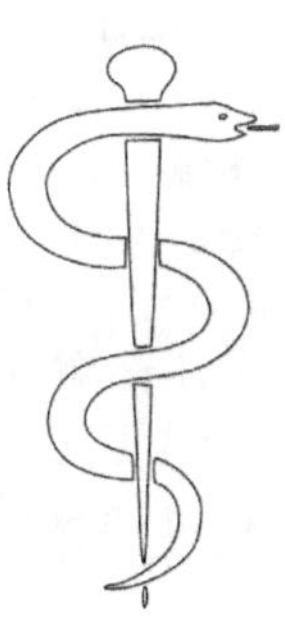

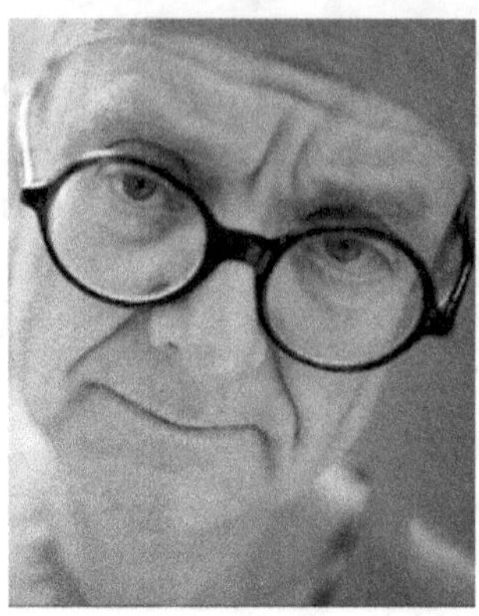

The Good, the Bad and the Ugly

No-one could see all 360 movies at the London Film Festival and whittling the choice down to less than a dozen is a challenge. You might begin by ruling out all the experimental films, the shorts, and the movies obviously aimed at niche audiences or with axes to grind. Then you learn to read between the lines of the eulogistic blurb which accompanies every offering. 'Slow burn' means the pace is glacial. 'Non-linear' means the story is incomprehensible to the audience and perhaps to the film-makers as well. 'Distinctive colour palate' means they couldn't afford in-date film. 'Restless camera' means you are likely to feel seasick. 'Coming of Age' –
well, you've lived it and seen it before.

Even then you can't win them all. I took my husband to see 10 ½ films. (The only thing that happened in the first 45 minutes of *Garage*, a vaguely distasteful film about a mentally slow garage hand, was that we walked out.) The other 10 films came from all over the world, and all were worth seeing. Three were particularly memorable.

The Good

The English Surgeon is a documentary about a neurosurgeon. All GPs know that surgeons are showmen, and that brain surgeons are ringmasters. Add charm and a dash of eccentricity and you have Henry Marsh, a neurosurgeon in south London.

Fifteen years ago Marsh went to Ukraine and met Igor Kurilets, a young doctor eager to set up a decent neurosurgical service in Kiev. Since then Marsh has been back many times and the film follows his visit to Ukraine last winter. He carried a suitcase full of tools of the trade which the NHS regards as disposable. In

Ukraine, where the primitive health facilities available to the poor drastically lengthen the odds against survival, they will save lives for many years to come. Against a bleak landscape (remind me never to visit Kiev in February) we find out how Igor Kurilets struggles against limited resources, old-fashioned attitudes to patients, government suspicion, inefficiency and professional jealousy. In such an atmosphere Henry Marsh's encouragement and moral support is as important as his practical help.

Kurilets has a list of cases he cannot tackle. Marsh is their only hope and they wait in the corridor, patient but desperate, for his judgement. We see one success – the removal of a brain tumour without anaesthetic – but what other doctors may find more moving is Marsh's visit to the family of a young girl he operated on some years ago. She died, but her family welcome Marsh and have laid on a feast to celebrate his visit. Being a successful doctor means failing sometimes, and this family understood that.

The film reminds us just how lucky we are in Britain, as doctors and as patients. The NHS is much better resourced, clinicians work together – mostly, patients are much more involved in what happens to them, the moral dilemmas are less stark. But Marsh, and the film, remind us that we cannot take any of this for granted. Ukraine's government appears not to understand doctors' altruism and patients' needs. Nor, it seems, does ours. Ukraine is slowly moving away from Stalinism in healthcare. Are we sliding towards it?

The Bad

Terror's Advocate (*L'Avocat de la Terreur*) is a chilling documentary. Jaques Vergès is a famous French lawyer. He came to notice when he defended, then married, then abandoned the Algerian terrorist Djamila Bouhired, who put a bomb in a milk bar which killed eleven people, and whose story was told in the film *The Battle of Algiers*. After disappearing for eight years Vergès returned to France, since when he has defended a long list of monsters including Nazi Klaus Barbie ('the butcher of Lyon'), Ilich Ramírez Sánchez (the terrorist known as 'Carlos the Jackal') and a string of Africa's more unsavoury dictators. He offered to defend Sadaam Hussein. Pol Pot, he feels, is much misunderstood.

He defends terrorists from the right and the left. "I would even defend George Bush, if he would plead guilty." His views are anti-colonialist – he is the son of a Vietnamese mother and Réunionese father, and France's colonial record is still a more inflammatory issue than Britain's. He is willing to challenge any state-held assumptions.

So far, perhaps so admirable, even if Vergès has pushed his self-assumed duty to an outrageous limit. But if you give someone enough rope they will hang themselves. Barbet Schroeder's film gives Vergès plenty of airtime to speak for himself. The result is a disquieting insight into the stunning egotism and chilling amorality of people who believe their ideas are worth more than other peoples' lives.

The Ugly

Life in the favelas of Rio de Janeiro was portrayed in *City of God*, and it is only marginally less ugly in *City of Men*. The plot (if you can follow it) is contrived, but it is only a peg on which to hang a picture of a world in which anarchy rules. The government has given up: schools, health care, rubbish collection don't seem to exist. Few people have jobs. Many have children, few children have a family. Rival gangs of young people, heavily armed and fuelled by drugs, are trapped in a never-ending chain of violent vengeance which destroys houses, homes and lives without thought and apparently without regret. Even the morality of gang loyalty is constantly breached.

Of course, there is always hope, even if just a crumb, and the film finds it in the last reel. But let us not be deceived; this is ugly and these days it is not so far from our own doorsteps. Though the brutish events of our inner-city ghettos are not played out against scenery as beautiful as the view from the favelas of Rio.

—NASGP February 2008

Photo: Henry Marsh

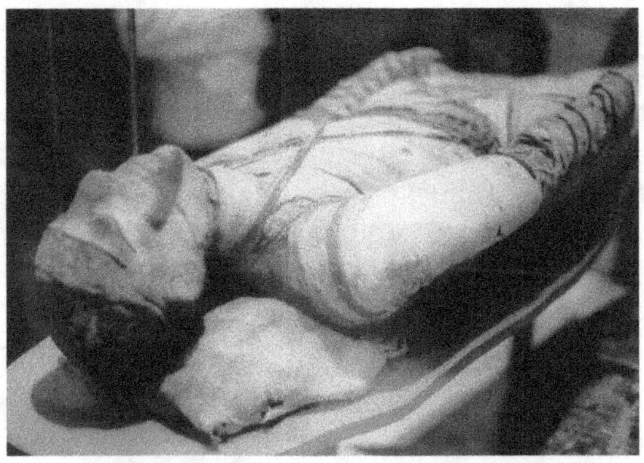

Return of the Mummy

Until 2004 it was illegal in this country to practise surgical techniques on cadavers. Dissection, yes, but not surgery. Throughout history attitudes to dead bodies have been shrouded in paradox. In every culture, the living invent rituals to appease the spirits of the dead.

Humans have been preserving their dead for 7,000 years. The ancient Egyptians did it so that the former owner's soul could recognise the body and inhabit it again in the afterlife. Pre-Inca customs in Peru probably had a similar purpose. In both areas the hot dry sand did a fairly good preservation job. Embalming appears to have evolved as a way to improve the prospects in the hereafter for those who could afford the expensive chemicals and rituals. The poor took their chances in the next world just as they did in this one.

Some things don't change: in California, cryonics now offers the very wealthy the hope of a future life, though not in the hereafter. Some modern embalming is less satisfactory in the long run. Just take a look at Lenin and Mao in their mausoleums.

The word mummy comes from the Persian *mummia*, for bitumen, which, mixed with spices, has been used since pharaonic times for preserving the bodies of the dead. Now, any body which is preserved from decomposition, whether it be by accident, like the occasional bog man, or deliberately, is called a mummy. But in most places stopping corpses from rotting is unrealistic. They have to be disposed of quickly by whatever means climate and terrain permit. Practicalities can change traditions: in Europe most religions have relaxed their bans on cremation. In India there are no longer enough vultures to devour the corpses on the Towers of

Silence, so the Parsi prohibition on burial is being lifted.

But, worldwide, the mystery of death demands rituals and the deceased's body must be treated with a dignity which respects its power. In medieval Britain denying a body burial in hallowed ground was a punishment; criminals' bodies were left on gibbets as a warning to the living. When anatomy became part of medical studies, a court could add the humiliation of subsequent dissection to a death sentence.

Come the Age of Enlightenment, more doctors and less capital punishment left anatomy schools undersupplied. Resurrection men filled the gap, digging up the recently deceased. In 1828 Burke and Hare sold the corpses of 16 people they had murdered to Edinburgh anatomist Dr Robert Knox. But public attitudes were slower to change. In 1788 poor New Yorkers rioted against the doctors and medical students whom they saw as responsible for the indignity visited upon their dead. The wealthy built elaborate fences and guards to protect the graves of their loved ones.

In the UK, the Anatomy Act of 1832 sought to meet the needs of the doctors and assuage the anxieties of the public: unclaimed and donated corpses could be dissected by licensed anatomy teachers. With the introduction of formaldehyde in 1867 cadavers lasted longer. The Human Tissue Act of 2004 permitted cadavers to be used for practising surgical techniques, but otherwise did not fundamentally change the law about dissection.

The public remains ambivalent about dead bodies. Egyptian mummies – cadavers, viewed from a safe distance in time – fascinated the Victorians. They held 'unwrapping parties' and shivered at the thought of the mummy's curse. In many parts of the world, body parts and fluids are still sold as cures. Even in the West we remain ambivalent: individuals, institutions and the law have been uneasy about anatomist Dr Gunter von Hagens' plastinated cadavers, but the public has flocked to his exhibitions, and the public autopsy he performed in 2002 attracted a lot of interest.

Modern techniques have also revolutionised medical training. The undergraduate initiation rite of the anatomy room is being swept away, more due to cost and doubts about its educational value than by sensitivity. Basic anatomy can be learned from virtual and plastinated bodies. But trainee surgeons cannot develop their skills on holograms, or even wax models. They need the real thing, or something very close. As anyone who did traditional anatomy remembers, bodies preserved in formaldehyde are unpleasant to work on and the flesh is stiff. But, using new methods of embalming like Theil soft fixing, tissues handle like living flesh. Now surgeons can gain useful experience without resorting to pigs. Or to us.

Now the mummy has returned. Four-thousand-year-old cadavers, however preserved, can now be subject to virtual autopsy. Using modern imaging and investigative techniques paleopathologists establish the age at death and often its cause, which has shaken a few myths. Ancient Egyptians had terrible dental health, not due to sugar but because the grit in milled cereals wore away their tooth enamel. Dental abscesses were very common – and must have been agonising. Atherosclerosis is not just a condition of our modern way of life: 35% of ancestral mummies from all over the world show evidence of it. So could there be a strong genetic element to ischaemic heart disease? Paleopathologists' studies of the cancers and mycobacteria from millennia ago shed light on the evolution of modern diseases and may contribute insights into how they may be managed in the 21st century.

Those ancient cultures that preserved their dead may not have ensured their everlasting life, but they are helping their modern descendants live better in this world.

—NASGP January 2015

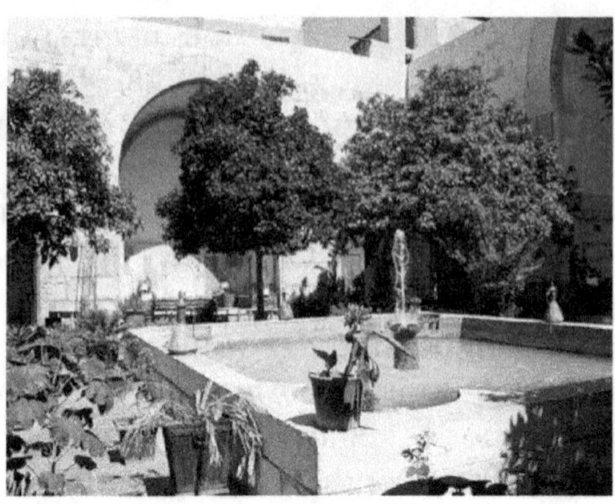

What Doctors Learned from the Arabs

Bashar Al-Assad was doing his specialist training in ophthalmology at the Western Eye Hospital in London when his brother Basil wrapped himself and his sports car round a tree. His father summoned Bashar back home to prepare to succeed him. When his father died in 2000, Bashar became president of Syria.

In Syria, Bashar's mild features gaze out from every shop window, every hoarding, even the rear windows of cars. It is said that he is temperamentally unsuited to dictatorship, but he has not managed to democratise his country and protests about the lack of freedom in Syria are being suppressed brutally, whether by his orders or those of his relatives who may exercise the real control. Bashar may be reflecting that, but for an RTA, he could be running a lucrative private practice, or, who knows, heading a national trachoma programme.

He came to London to learn from the medical expertise of the West and take it back to Syria. But a thousand years ago the traffic of medical knowledge was all the other way.

At school I had to memorise a list of 'Things we learned from the Arabs'. It included algebra and the silver-coated pill. I rather wished that we had not learned algebra, and I had never seen a silver-coated pill and did not see why merely adding silver to a pill should make it more effective. It took many years – till last month – for me to find out what the Arabs did know about medicine.

The Maristan in Damascus was built as a medical school in 1154 by Sultan Nur Ad-Din, and remained active as a hospital until the 19th century. The elegant building is now a medical museum, and it is possible to sit and relax in one of the *iwans* – the vaulted recesses off the courtyard where consultations and lessons were held – admiring the fountain and the display of medicinal plants, and reflecting on the sophistication of medical knowledge developed in this part of the world. It gradually filtered to the West, much of it probably translated into Latin or directly into Castilian at the school of translators in Toledo, Spain.

On display in the old wards there are remarkably modern-looking diagrams of the structure of the eye and the heart. Types of facial paralysis, and symptoms and complications of diabetes are described. They knew about the infective nature of TB centuries before it was accepted in the West. Damascene doctors had charts to check which herbs and preparations were useful for what conditions. Dried lizard as an aphrodisiac might not pass the evidence-based medicine test (though I guess some wouldn't mind being enrolled in a trial), but many preparations are still in use today, in allopathic as well as complementary practice. And like modern doctors, they sometimes called on a bit of magic as well, if the basket of talismans is anything to go by.

I thought Dr John Snow developed inhalational anaesthesia in the 19th century. At the Maristan Nur Ad-Din you can see the sponge that doctors there used centuries earlier to administer a mixture of hashish, opium and belladonna dissolved in alcohol to surgical patients. Like Snow, they challenged the belief that pain is the price we pay for mankind's sins.

Al-Zawhrawi's dentist's chair has a neck support and a ratchet for tipping back the head. He filled teeth with gold and silver, and saw extractions as a failure. Not surprising, except that this dentist died in 1013.

It is clear that the relationship between physical and mental health was understood. The Bimaristan Arghoun al-Kamili in Aleppo cared for patients with mental health problems from its founding (with a grant for research) in 1354 until the 20th century. Like Nur Ad-Din's hospital in Damascus, it offered patients an environment designed to rehabilitate them. Patients had rooms around a series of courtyards and the sound and sight of the fountain at the centre of each courtyard was an important part of their therapy. The courtyard for the most seriously disturbed patients has small rooms, barred for safety and rather dark because it was believed that low light levels were soothing, but patients could hear and see the fountain, and they were given a healthy diet and calming herbal teas.

As patients improved they moved to open rooms around a larger courtyard and were allowed out to sit in the *iwan* and listen to musicians playing round the fountain. There was a separate courtyard for female patients. On discharge all patients were given money for clothes and food to tide them over till they could work for themselves.

It is salutary to reflect that in Britain at that time, people with psychiatric conditions were locked up and chained, or drowned or burned as witches, and in Russia last century political dissidents were confined under brutal conditions in mental hospitals. It is to be hoped that President Assad will treat his people with the wisdom and understanding that his forbears 1,000 years ago showed to their patients.

—NASGP June 2011

POSTSCRIPT (March 2015*):* A lot has happened since I was in Syria four years ago, none of it good. People I met have been abducted and almost certainly brutally murdered, historic sites have been severely damaged and the medieval souk in Aleppo where people still did most of their shopping has been largely destroyed, and with it probably the hospital I describe in the article.

Photo: First Courtyard, Maristan Nur ad-Din, Damascus, 2011

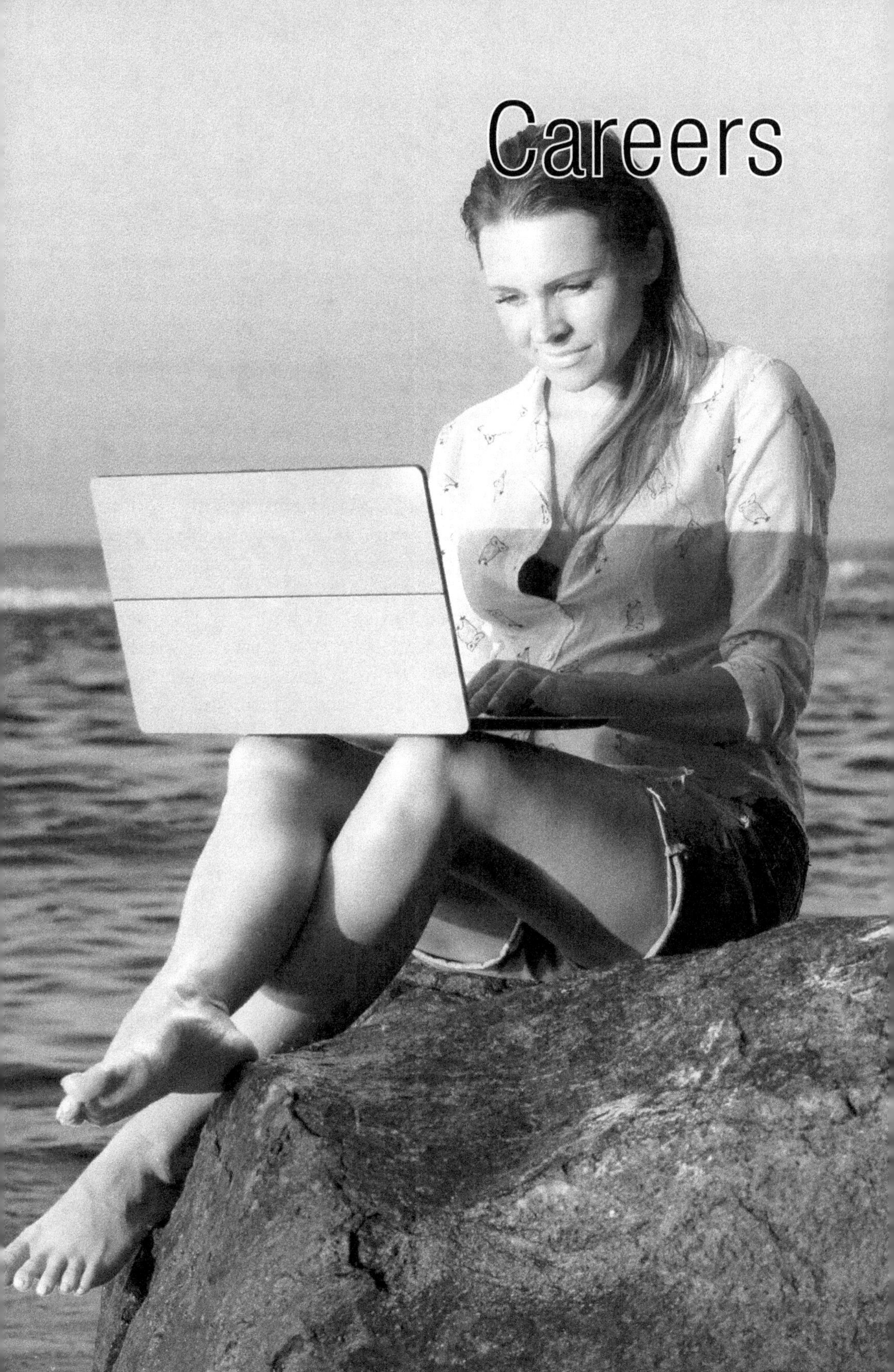

Careers

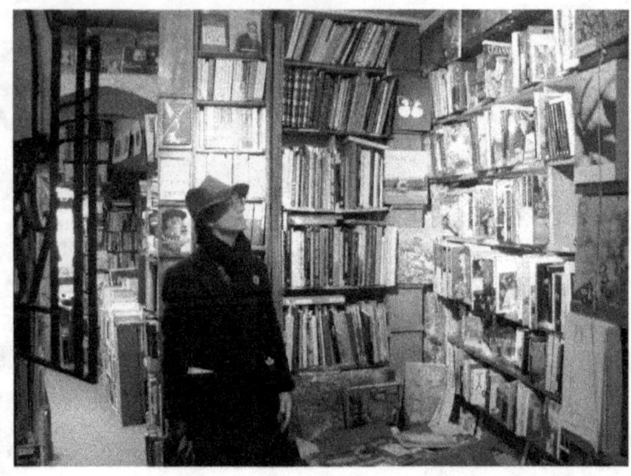

A la Recherche du Temps Perdu

I have just been clearing out old textbooks, cuttings from Update and BMJ from the days before information could be stored electronically, even some old lecture notes (did I once know all that?).

Since I don't recall my days as a clinical student with fondness, I was surprised while leafing through dog-eared volumes to feel a degree of nostalgia, though not strongly enough to put many books back on the shelf. However, a few escaped the cull.

I couldn't bring myself to throw away my first *Oxford Handbook of Clinical Medicine*. The first edition came out just in time for my house-jobs, and it kept me sane and my patients safe. Well, safer. In those days the recto pages of Oxford handbooks were blank, for you to make your own notes. Invaluable for recording the sort of clinical gems which evidence-based medicine cannot reach. They were useful too for noting that consultant A wanted all patients admitted with diagnosis B to be put on drug C, whereas consultant D would tear you off a strip if he saw C on a patient's drug chart.

Looking at my annotations took me back to Treliske Hospital in the middle of a summer night. GPs calling from remote villages with long Cornish names. Sick patients admitted from holiday cottages proud to be on some 'very special pills' from a professor in the Midlands who has instructed them they 'must never stop them', but unable to remember what the pills were. The lack of space in the admissions unit. The lack of beds in the hospital. Trying to grab a few minutes of rest curled up on two chairs. The naval helicopter from Culdrose bringing in a Bulgarian seaman winched off a Russian ship in the Bay of Biscay. They hadn't winched off his medical history and it took some time before a

Russian speaker was tracked down in Falmouth. Vivid memories of an important six months.

I slipped two other books back on the shelf. Both are slim. One I kept because it is both dated and dateless. Dated because of the black-and-white photographs. The headless torso of a man in a long white coat buttoned across a middle-aged corporation and revealing only his tie demonstrates the muscle groups on a discretely photographed colleague, supplemented by diagrams of the brachial plexus (did I ever know that?) and the lateral cutaneous nerve of the thigh (why do I remember that?). Dateless because it is a guide to neuroanatomy, and neuroanatomy does not change. Do they still hand out *Aids to the Examination of the Peripheral Nervous System* (Her Majesty's Stationery Office, £1.75) on Day One of the anatomy course? Do they still have anatomy courses?

The second book is also a neurology *aide memoire*, and it was a chance finding. I was in a New York bookshop, flicking through books on how to get into medical school, how to survive once you got there, how to pass finals and how to survive once you had done so, and reflecting on what wimps American medical students must be, when a title caught my eye. *Clinical Neuroanatomy Made Ridiculously Simple*. What a promise! And it was written by a professor from a medical school in Miami. If they could understand it in Florida, perhaps I could! I snapped it up and could have made a tidy income importing copies for resale to my fellow students because Blackwell's bookshop didn't stock it. Sir Basil Blackwell would have set his face adamantly against dumbing down. But they stock it now. The cover is unchanged and though it's in its 3rd edition the evolution seems to be not anatomical but technological – it is now interactive, whatever that means. Amazon gives it five-star reviews from UK students.

In years to come will doctors who are now at the start of their careers look back fondly on *gpnotebook.co.uk* and treasure the URL of *Map of Medicine*? It seems unlikely. Does it matter? Perhaps. As you grow older, you lose touch with your younger self, and while you don't want to know how they treated SLE in 1982 and may prefer not to recall what you got up to at the post-finals party, a textbook can retrieve long-buried memories. And give you back a part of yourself.

—NASGP June 2010

Photo: The author in Shakespeare and Company, Paris

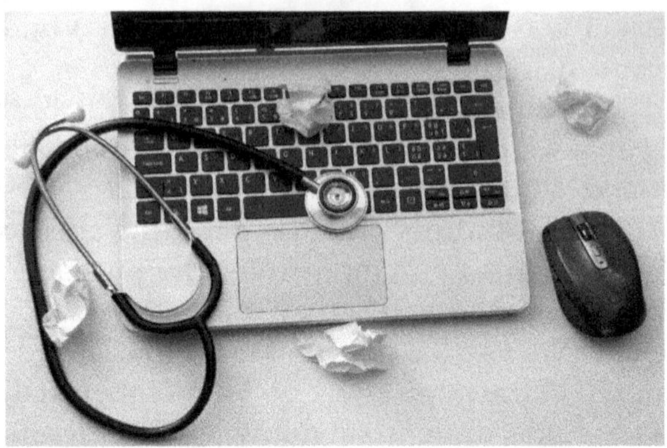

GP Locums: Who Wouldn't Want to Be One?

Good locums are never short of work because they have special skills. Walking into an unknown practice to see 30 unknown patients and departing four hours later, leaving not only those patients but also the staff with positive impressions, is a challenge. But for those who can develop the flexibility, being a locum is not just satisfying, it offers an interesting way of life.

Locums forgo the traditional reward of general practice, the long-term relationship that GPs develop with patients. Patients rarely choose to see a locum.

So the task is to make the 10 minutes that you and a patient spend together rewarding for both of you. You can give patients the opportunity to tell their story afresh. At least you can offer a new view of an old problem. Perhaps you will spot a missed diagnosis.

Locums are never – well, rarely – bored. Is the surgery full of patients expecting antibiotics for a cold? Perhaps you can change the culture of the practice and persuade at least some of them there is no magic bullet for viral illnesses. Struggling with a badly organised practice? Can you find an acceptable way to offer advice so that when you or a colleague next work there, things function a little better? Is the clinical care substandard, even dangerous? Dealing with colleagues' incompetence is not easy, but it is a professional obligation and potentially saves more lives than all the statins you will ever prescribe.

Not being tied to a practice has advantages. Unlike a partner, you can walk away from a practice you never want to work in again. Managing practices in the 21st-century NHS is increasingly onerous. Locums do not have to do it – you can concentrate on patient care. Nor do locums have to negotiate holidays with three other partners with school-aged children. You are your own boss. This has its own responsibilities, but allows you to devote more time to seeing patients and you can more easily fit work around family and other commitments. Take a holiday any time you wish.

Being a locum combines well with a portfolio career. Work as a GP three days a week and as a dermatologist or a tree surgeon on the other two. Or spend six months as a full-time GP in the UK and six months with Médecins Sans Frontières in Angola. You can even drop out to climb in the Andes, fence in the Olympics or write your novel without fractious negotiation with partners about time off. True, you will not be paid if you stop work to have a baby or study law, but if you plan your finances carefully, you can make space in your life for anything you want to do.

If you are a newly qualified GP, you may envy friends who move straight into partnership. But they miss the opportunity to broaden their experience. You may be a locum because there is nothing else available, but make the most of it. If you have spent your time so far in suburbia, try a taste of the inner city, or head for the hills to sample rural practice. You can try big and small practices, practices designed for the homeless, practices with traditional lists and those where part-time GPs see most patients.

You can come to grips with different medical software and different ways of recording consultations. Is nurse triage as good as doctor triage? How can a practice ensure safe handover? Is treating diseases of the rich appealing, or do you prefer to confront the problems of the poor? You can try out practices to see if you would like a salaried post or partnership there. You will have a range of models to draw on in designing your career and later on being a locum can be a rewarding way to wind down to retirement.

For practices in a jam, a locum is a lifesaver. Being welcomed by a practice with a doctor off sick and a waiting room full of patients is a good start to the day, and leaving with thanks ringing in your ears is a great goodbye. It is nice to be needed, and good locums always are.

—A version of this article first appeared on www.gponline.com in 2011

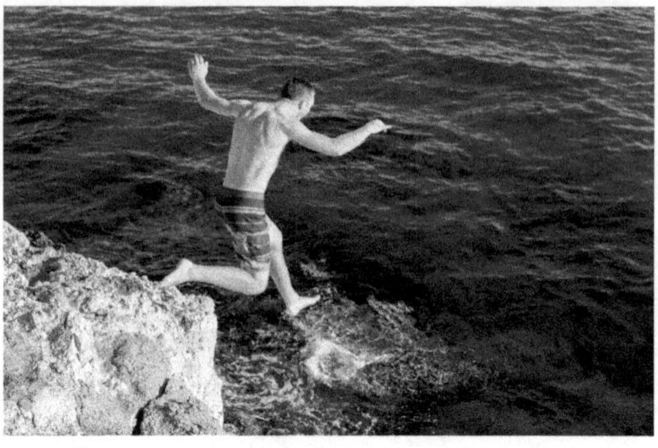

GP Locums: It's a Riskier Job

GPs live with risk. It is what we do every day when deciding which treatment options are the best for our patients. Being a locum ups the stakes, but the risk level can be managed.

Allowing yourself to be logged into practices' clinical systems as 'locum' rather than with your own unique log-in is akin to a warning siren, because the resulting audit trails are open to challenge.

Never undertake something beyond your competence. Just say "no". It is better to clarify the practice's expectations by agreeing a job description in advance. Use a booking form: the National Association of Sessional GPs (NASGP) has a standard one. Otherwise, you may arrive on a bicycle and find you are expected to visit a patient on a remote farm.

Be alert to being 'forced to underperform'. If the practice's urine test strips are out of date and it does not have a pulse oximeter, your best may not be good enough.

I set out for my first morning as a locum with a stethoscope and diagnostic set in my handbag. Two days later, I had a backpack with sphygmomanometer, peak flow meter, thermometer, tape measure, drugs directory and in-date dipsticks. And I know locums who wheel suitcases containing laptop, printer and dictating machine.

Then there are the insidious, harder-to-avoid and more difficult-to-manage risks you cannot put on a tick list.

Time pressure is one. Everything takes longer if you are new to a practice, and running behind puts you under pressure. That is when doctors make mistakes. You are not listening as carefully or thinking as clearly as normal.

You are tempted to cut corners. And the longer your patients have been waiting, the worse you feel and the less forgiving they are if they think something has gone wrong.

This is challenging if, like me, you are a slow consulter. Seek help. Discuss the problem with fellow locums. Video some consultations and ask a GP tutor for advice on consulting more quickly but effectively.

Then there are the attempts to exploit your goodwill. We all want to receive grateful thanks from practices. But treat requests such as "Could you possibly . . . ?" and "Would you mind just . . . for me?" as red flags.

Can you really safely squeeze in a patient who arrived late? Should you comment on an X-ray report pushed under your nose between consultations because the patient is creating hell at the front desk?

Handover is another bear trap. Ask what the practice's handover system is, and add a belt if the braces seem frayed. Remember that handwritten notes can get lost. For example, the receptionist who promised to pass on information goes off sick. The secretary, like you, is only temporary and leaves your letter in a heap as she assumes you will be in tomorrow to sign it.

Do not be afraid to duplicate information about a patient whose condition worries you. If your note fails to reach the right person at the right time, this could cost the patient their life and you, your career.

Signing repeat prescriptions is a minefield. Partners may be happy to scribble signatures on a thick pile in 10 minutes, but as a locum, you need to look at the patients' notes – especially if you suspect the practice's repeat prescribing policy is not robust enough.

Life is risky, so analyse the dangers and do what you can to reduce them.

—A version of this article first appeared on www.gponline.com in 2011

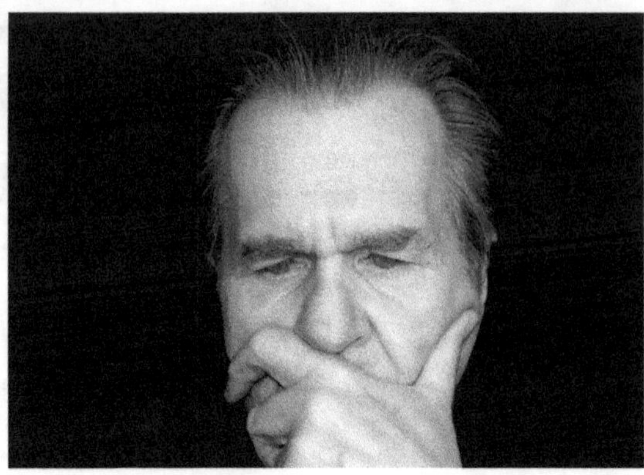

GP Locums: When to Blow the Whistle?

Should you blow the whistle if you suspect a practice is failing? As a locum, you are in a very strong position. Sitting in colleagues' rooms, reading their patients' notes and using their equipment means you see practices from the inside.

You are also in a very weak position. You are isolated. If you encounter something worrying, then wondering whether you are justified in bringing it to someone's attention can make you feel very vulnerable.

The ethical position is clear. The GMC's Good Medical Practice places a professional obligation on doctors to put the safety of patients first.

A locum has to address anything that could put a patient at risk. It might be the practice's building: fire exits blocked or unshielded electrical sockets into which toddlers could push their fingers.

It might be equipment: no foetal heart rate monitor, broken sphygmomanometers. It might be systems: no review dates for repeat medications, no security protocol for faxes.

It might be staff: doctors prescribing steroid drops for red eyes and antibiotics for everyone, receptionists issuing prescriptions without a doctor's agreement.

The responsibility can feel daunting, but you are not alone. Bad practice is not rare and so there are plenty of people and organisations to advise and support you. Plug the number of your defence organisation into your phone. Don't be afraid to ring them, however trivial the query may seem. That is why you pay that large subscription fee.

And join your local sessional GP group. Then, when you need peer support, you have people you know to turn to.

So, if you reach the end of your session with concerns about something at the practice, what steps should you take?

If you spot something minor in a generally good practice – for example, a wobbly stool, which sooner or later will tip a patient onto the floor as they climb on to the couch – a tactful word with the practice manager before you leave is probably all that is needed to ensure the problem is remedied. Check next time you work there, or ask a colleague to do so.

At the other extreme, if you think a patient's life is in danger or you suspect a criminal offence, do not delay. Ring your defence organisation before you leave the practice

Most concerns fall between these extremes: the questionable prescription, the investigation that apparently has not been followed up. There could be an innocent explanation.

It is tempting to downplay your concerns. But remember your professional obligation. Your defence organisation will guide you through what you should do next. It can advise on how to validate your observations, whom to contact about your concern, how the practice should be informed that questions have been raised about it, whether a patient should be notified and, if so, by whom.

Your sessional GP group provides a safe, confidential discussion forum. Some colleagues may have worked at the practice and share your anxiety. Even if no-one else has seen anything amiss, in future they will be alert to problems.

Remember too that LMC Secretaries have a shrewd idea of the standard of local practices and want to know if colleagues' or practices' performance is giving cause for concern.

The primary care organisation (PCO) is responsible for the safety of patients in its area. Your defence organisation can advise you on involving the PCO, whom to contact and what to say. The PCO's medical director or clinical governance lead are the usual channels, but there may be more appropriate points of contact.

Resist the temptation to trawl for evidence to support your suspicions. By accepting the job you agreed to the practice's policy on use of their data, and taking a screenshot or photographing the notes puts you in the wrong. Nor do you want to have to hand over your mobile phone laden with confidential data. Once you have reported your concerns, it is not up to you to provide proof.

Blowing the whistle is never easy. If you are suffering sleepless nights, seek help. The BMA's *Doctors For Doctors* service is a confidential helpline. If you are desperate, a trained counsellor is on the end of the phone 24 hours a day.

If you need peer support, the service will give you a telephone appointment with a doctor adviser. An independent colleague can be easier to talk to than someone you know.

If you ever feel tempted to persuade yourself that there was not really a problem, consider two things.

Firstly, even if the practice has provided you with out-of-date test strips, if you miss a patient's raised blood sugar and the patient suffers as a result, you are responsible.

Secondly, how would you feel if the patient were your mother?

—A version of this article first appeared on www.gponline.com in 2011

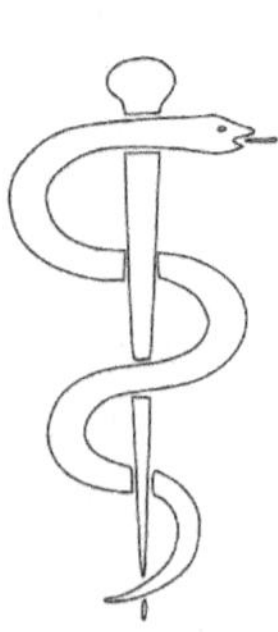

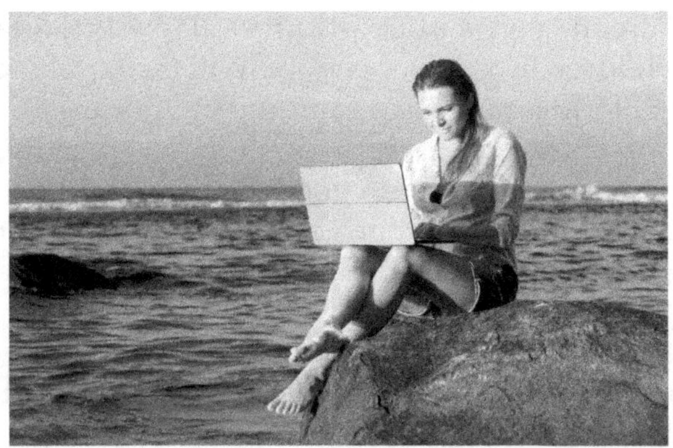

GP Locums: It's a Tough Balancing Act

Surely being a GP locum is all about doing a few weeks' work, charging megabucks to do surgeries and then zooming off as an expedition doctor, watching wildlife in Africa while treating the odd case of sunburn.

In your dreams. True, GP locums have flexibility, but as most quickly realise, flexibility comes at a price. GP partners and salaried GPs are buffered by the structure of the practice while GP locums have to manage everything for themselves.

GP locums, like all self-employed people, all too often work when they would be better off home in bed, or at least with their feet up resting. Under pressure to fulfil commitments and to pay the mortgage, we exempt ourselves from the counsel we offer patients. And the cost can be to our long-term health.

Probably the most important step a GP locum can take to maintain a healthy work-life balance is to do a personal audit. And like all audits, it is only useful if it is acted upon and repeated at intervals.

Sit down and ask yourself some basic questions. Involve your family; their quality of life is at stake as well as yours. What are your financial needs now and in the foreseeable future? How do you see your career developing and what are your ambitions, both professional and personal?

How much money do you need? And how does this translate into hours of work per week, month or year? Is such a workload sustainable? If not, how can you increase your rates or cut your costs?

You may need to prioritise income generation for a while, but set limits. And if you are continually in danger of toppling over the financial cliff, revise your priorities. How important is it to send your children to private schools? Will the family really enjoy a holiday in Florida more than camping in France?

Beware of conscience creep: don't allow pleading practice managers to manipulate your good nature. Build time off into your schedule. Make sure that you block off important days so you don't miss seeing your daughter in the school play or your son scoring a hat-trick.

Build gaps into your schedule to spend quality time with your family – there is no point working full-out to retirement and then regretting missing your children's defining moments.

Build in holidays. Ring fence these areas as rigorously as the royal enclosure at Ascot. And if your family complain that it doesn't see enough of you, look for something you all enjoy together. Whether this is going to the local swimming pool or doing jigsaws, it doesn't matter as long as everyone has fun.

Insurance is important to peace of mind, but it always seems very expensive, until you need to call on it. Then it is worth every penny. Sure, if you could bear the cost of triplets, don't pay to insure yourself against multiple births. But if an accident or chronic illness would leave you and your family struggling financially, you need to protect against the risk

Invest in your health, and heed your GP's advice and your own common sense. If you are not well, don't work. Other GPs at the practice can cover for a GP off sick, but GP locums have to be on top form every session they work.

Doctors who are unwell make more mistakes. And it is not just patients' health which is at risk. It's your health and your career too.

Burnout is a common problem. 'Rustout' (boredom at work) is also corrosive to happiness. If you are exhausted or bored how can you revive yourself?

A new professional interest perhaps. There are plenty of opportunities: teaching, medical politics or learning a new clinical skill, for example. Or a hobby.

Do something creative (interpret this broadly), which gives you back some of what medicine takes out of you. And you don't want to reach retirement wondering what might have been. So if you have a desire to work in the Australian outback or play the cello or climb K2, start planning now.

As a GP locum, you have to shoulder the personal administration of your career, which partners are spared, more or less, because there is the practice manager and practice accountant to look after most of it for you.

But even GP locums can delegate. Is there a GP locum chambers near you, or could you start one? A chambers gives you not only administrative and financial back-up but also colleagues.

Isolation is a threat to locums and if your work-life balance is out of kilter, colleagues offer a sounding board and a way of recalibrating yourself. If you are persistently at the wrong end of the bell-shaped satisfaction curve, you need to take action. A mentor could help you tilt your life back into balance.

Like everything else in a locum's life, achieving a satisfying work-life balance is no-one's responsibility but yours, and it is in your hands. It's your life and happiness, and your family's too. It's worth working at.

—A version of this article first appeared on www.gponline.com in 2011

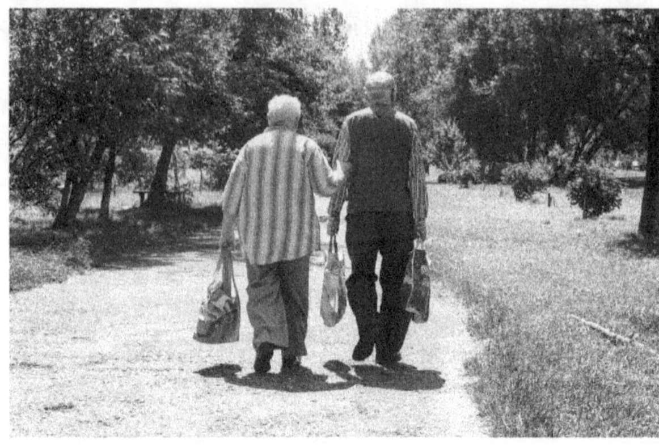

Planning Your Exit Strategy

The only certainties in life, said Benjamin Franklin, are death and taxes. As GPs we see the infirmities and indignities of old age, but we probably suppress the knowledge that in time we will be similarly afflicted. Yet we may well live a quarter century or more after retirement. Old age encroaches slowly but it always comes as a surprise. And no-one can look back on old age. So we don't have a guidebook to help us through it. Planning your exit strategy is even less fun than planning your pension, but it's just as important.

Here are some thoughts we could be putting to our patients, and to ourselves as we move into middle age.

- However bad your health, remember that living to old age is a privilege. And better than the alternative. Find one thing a day to treasure, however small, whether it's a walk among the bluebells, or just a bird on the windowsill.

- At retirement, most people still have plenty of energy. Maintain your old interests and friendships, but invest in new activities which you can continue as you age. Whether you go for learning Chinese or china-mending or growing prize dahlias, you will keep your mind alive, and you will meet people. Something that attracts a wide age group allows you to develop relationships with younger people, especially valuable when your peers start dropping away. Your contemporaries can sympathise with your painful feet; younger people can help you forget them.

- Build up social credit while you can. There are plenty of opportunities to be useful after retirement. If you have helped others, if you have been a life-enhancer, if you have been a good friend, you will have people who are happy to offer help when you need it.

- Use it or lose it. Regular exercise maintains muscle strength and balance and mental well-being. And if your press-up days are well behind you, you can still walk, shuffle or even Zimmer down to the post-box on the corner. No matter that you don't have a letter to post, the fresh air and exercise will invigorate your muscles, your bowels and your mind.

- If you can't get out, do what you can to avoid becoming chair-shaped. Even just standing up for a few minutes once an hour will help.

- Keep things clean. If you live alone it is easy to let things go, especially if you are depressed or tired or have limited mobility or can't see the mould on the bread. But it's dispiriting to visit someone who hasn't washed or cleaned their teeth for a week, who is sitting in grubby clothes on a stained chair surrounded by biscuit crumbs and dusty piles of old magazines. Even if you can't afford home help, be determined to keep up standards.

- De-clutter your life and your home. Don't leave decisions about what happens to your mementoes and tea-spoon collection to your executors. As eastern religions recognise, getting rid of possessions is liberating.

- Beware the chains of routine. Be as flexible as you can in habit as well as body. If someone offers to take you out for tea, don't decline because you always have your hair done on Tuesday afternoons.

- When someone phones, never, ever, say "It's so nice to hear a human voice". It puts such a responsibility on your caller. If you haven't spoken to anyone for a week, ring someone you know. Check that it's convenient for them to chat, and if it isn't arrange a time.

- It's tempting to rely on your children to meet all your physical and emotional needs, but it isn't fair. Try not to leave anyone with the awful burden of feeling that you are totally dependent on them.

- Keep up with the latest IT for as long as you can. Today's elderly who can use email are able to maintain contacts and manage their lives, even though their hearing makes phone-calls tricky and their Parkinson's makes writing difficult and verbal arrangements fall through gaps in their memory. Who knows how people will communicate in the future, but it is important that when we are elderly, *we* know how.

- Have things to talk about. You don't need to go to a football match, or to a Tracey Emin exhibition, to have an opinion. Again, being IT-savvy is important. If you can find your way round the web, your TV or tomorrow's gadget, you can keep up with the outside world and contribute to discussions. Don't leave learning new ways till it's too late; get into audio books, DVDs by post, music downloads while it's easy to learn.
- There are lots of books about how to be young, but Diana Athill's *Somewhere Towards the End* is one of the few about how to be old. At 94, she has had time to think about it. Two pieces of her advice: it's useless to fret over regrets; and ordinary things become precious when you know you won't be able to enjoy them much more. So make the most of every day.

📖 ***Somewhere Towards the End*** *Diana Athill, 2008*

—NASGP April 2012

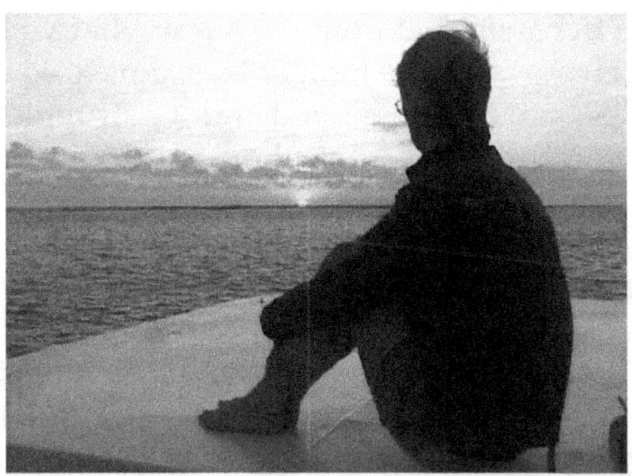

Giving Up . . . or Stopping?

When I first became a GP, there was a problem with easing octogenarians out of the practices they had served for more than half a century. Then came Mrs Thatcher's purchaser-provider split and a new GP contract. Suddenly grey-haired GPs became an endangered species and no-one wanted to go into general practice. Now in 2007 there are not enough openings to go round for newly trained GPs, and their older colleagues seem to be finding more options for the last years of their working lives.

NASGP's membership includes doctors of all ages. There are will-be partners, have-been partners, may-be partners and won't-be partners. I fall into the second category, and like many colleagues have found that flexibility as a sessional or freelance GP has returned to me control over my work and my life, and restored my enjoyment in seeing patients. It has been a great six years.

Now I am about to give up. "NO!" said a friend who has already done so. "We are not giving up, we are stopping." We doctors have a strong tendency to do guilt, and if you were lucky enough to secure a place to train as a mature student, as I was, you have even more to beat yourself up over. But we should not apologise when we recognise that it is time to move on.

GPs are used to change. After all, each working day we start again every ten minutes. And we are constantly learning to keep up with new drugs, techniques, new ways of doing things. Change keeps you flexible, keeps you young. Until it wears you out. It's not what you do; that changes slowly. It's not patients who change. Their problems and worries have as much to do with the human condition – unchanging – as with disease, and even disease doesn't change that much. It's not what you do, it's how you do it that changes. At the moment it seems to change monthly. 'DESs' and 'LISs' are commissioned and we struggle to remember what codes we are to use, then they are decommissioned and that doesn't count any more. Every time there is a reorganisation some doctors, usually those towards the end of their careers, will call it a day. Been there, done that twenty years ago and it didn't work then. When you have got to the stage in life where one new fact inserted into the brain pushes one old fact out, you quickly feel overloaded. When I give up – sorry, stop – I look forward to getting my brain back. I think of all that space which will be available for all the things that over the years have been stuffed into the cramped corners of my cerebrum.

Will I miss it? Yes, of course. The multitude of human contacts, the fascination of the glimpse into other people's lives, the intellectual stimulation are addictive. But there are other things to do and new pleasures to be found.

I'm not giving up. I'm stopping. And starting again.

—*NASGP October 2007*

Photo: En route to the Galapagos

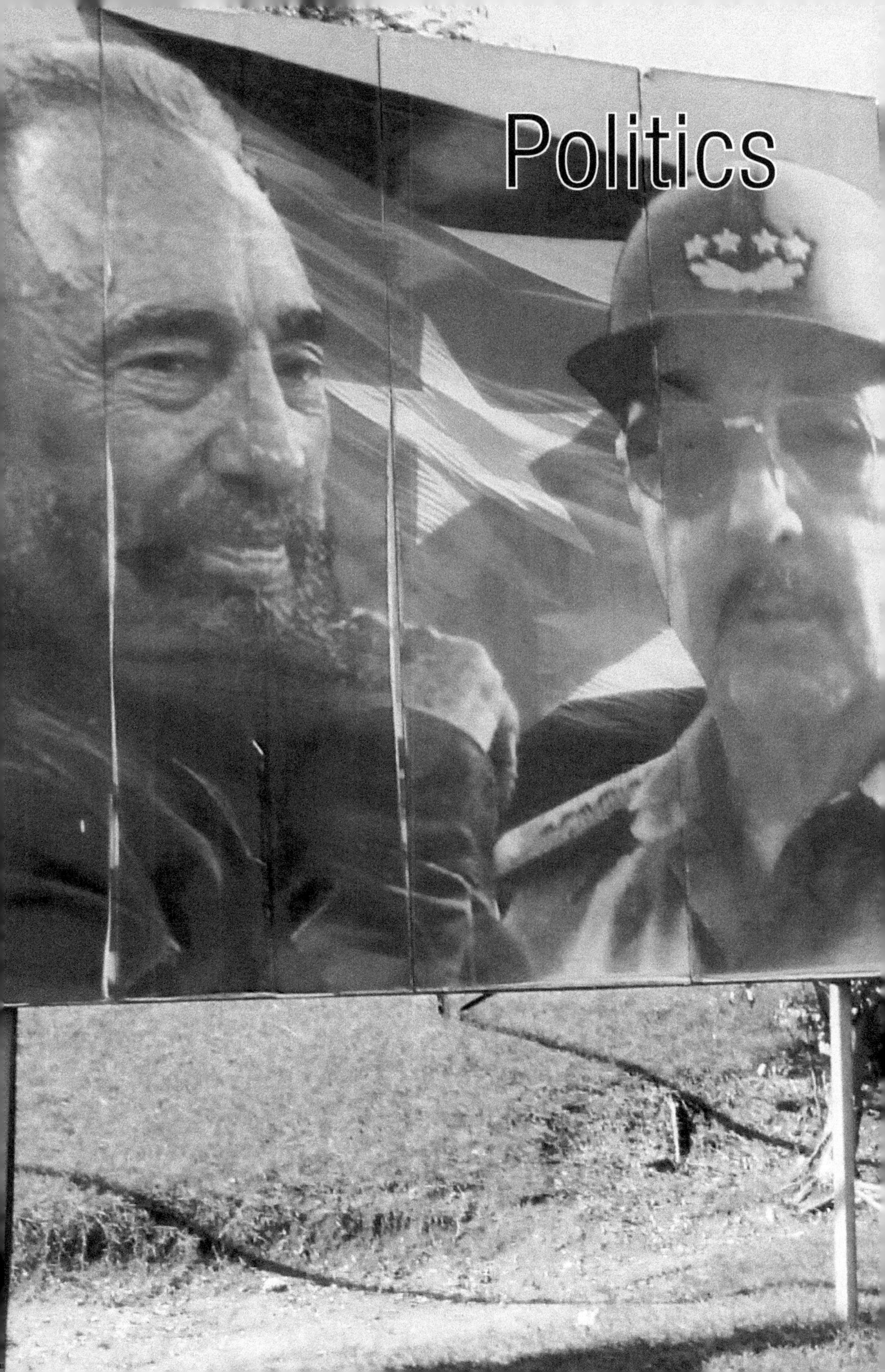
Politics

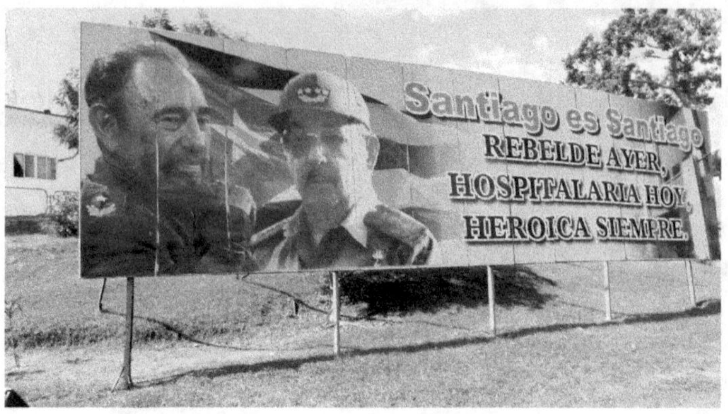

Are We Still All Right, Jack?

Around the middle of the 20th century three countries introduced systems designed to provide primary health care to all their citizens: the UK, China and Cuba. All three nations had emerged from devastating conflicts with a political commitment to more equal societies. All achieved success in reducing health inequalities. Through universally applied public health programmes, education, and free family health care, each country combated the ravages of infectious diseases and ignorance, lowered childhood mortality and improved the expectation of life.

Half a century later, China's barefoot doctors are a distant memory. In the UK the social contract that underpins the NHS is under threat. Only Cuba has kept the faith, to the advantage of the health of its citizens who enjoy a first world expectation of life for a third world cost.

When I worked for VSO in 1970s, Mao's barefoot doctor system was the model for provision of healthcare in poor countries. Villagers, sometimes traditional herbalists, were given simple training and with the support of their communes provided free basic personal and public health care to their communities. The evidence is that it worked.

Fast forward 30 years: a few months ago a young doctor from Shanghai spent a morning in practice with me learning about our primary health care system. I enquired about barefoot doctors. She looked at me as if I had asked about sending boy sweeps up chimneys. "That was before I was born!" she said.

What happened? Barefoot doctors acquired shoes and aspirations, costs increased, and within 20 years the Chinese people were again having to pay for healthcare. Which means that millions of people, particularly in rural areas, now go without.

In the UK, the NHS still functions, in some ways very well, in other ways poorly. Most patients are appreciative of the service they receive, in fact more appreciative than the government wishes to acknowledge.

In Britain, health is a political football. One could not claim that health in Cuba is not a political issue. Everything in Cuba is a political issue. But you cannot play football when there is just one team on the field. So the Cuban game is not driven by political point-scoring. Cuba's healthcare system has evolved, but in response to need not to politics.

Political stability must help to maintain a vision. So must social stability. Britain's population, the way we live and the way we earn our living – or don't – has changed a lot since the NHS was founded. If in doubt, take a look at films like *I'm All Right Jack*. In contrast, Cuba today probably doesn't look so different from the early Castro years. For better or for worse. It is still dependent on sugar. There is very little traffic on the roads. True, tourism, so much a feature of the Batista era, is back, along with some of the old blights such as prostitution, but today's package visitors are largely corralled on cayes which ordinary Cubans may only visit if they are employed there. For better or worse.

But there has to be more to Cuba's achievements than that. The answer may lie in just what has made the NHS so popular and cost-effective: a family doctor system which puts the relationship between doctor and patients at the heart of the health of the community. Though Cuban family doctors have a stronger remit than UK GPs to promote healthy living. I wonder how many British GPs have taken a look in a patient's fridge to check on their diet, or led their patients in exercise classes?

It may be that the US embargo fosters a shared self-help ethos in Cuba, and undoubtedly the absence of McDonalds and prudent use of scarce foodstuffs contributes to health. Just as blockade, rationing and digging for victory did in wartime Britain.

In Britain, governments are trying to make health another commodity. But it isn't a commodity. Good health is a privilege; it requires some luck and a modest amount of work, and the optimism to make the best of what you have. We GPs are privileged to accompany and advise our patients on their road through life. Surely we don't need a Blitz mentality to preserve this?

—NASGP January 2008

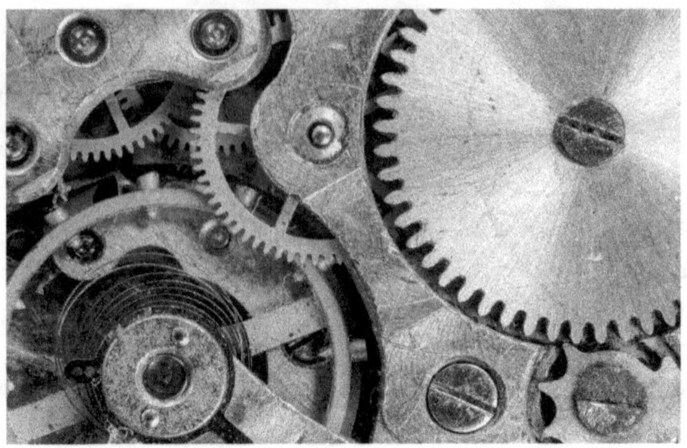

When Efficiency Is Ineffective

Everyone knows the NHS is inefficient. Lost X-rays, long waits for someone in a hospital to answer their phone or find the doctors on call, wasted medication. Even general practice is far from 100% efficient.

'Efficiency savings' are demanded as if they were achievable and free of downsides. But it is a weasel term. Even if someone realises that for thirty-five years secretaries have been obeying an ordnance to generate and file seven copies of every letter they type, how much will be saved by reducing the copies to one? How many repeat X-rays do you have to avoid to save half a million pounds? The sad truth is that the easiest way to cut expenditure, especially in the timescale demanded by politicians, is to cut services. In practice, 'efficiency savings' mean cuts in the budget for clinical care.

Efficiency isn't an absolute. It depends on your viewpoint. If you spend half an hour waiting to see your GP, that's inefficient for you. But 100% efficiency for every patient – no wait for the doctor – would require many more doctors who would spend much of their time twiddling their thumbs. Everyone pays for that inefficiency. So there is almost always a trade-off. But every so often, someone who doesn't work at the coal face of patient care thinks they have identified a wasteful practice and decides they can make the system more efficient. Accountants calculate that porters are only pushing trolleys 80% of the time so rule that the hospital can manage with 20% fewer porters. Try it and the hospital seizes up. The person – or committee – that proposed that every patient in the country wanting a GP appointment with their GP should ring a central number didn't have a clue. The surgeries would fill up with heartsink patients and the worried well. Good receptionists use their knowledge of patients, and their families and even their pets, to calm the distressed, to divine the importance of the problem and to steer patients to the right appointment. The call centre idea was quickly shelved.

There are plenty of politicians and managers who think that efficiency and effectiveness are the same thing. The truth is we live in an inefficient universe. Even the best machine is far from 100% efficient, whether it be man-made or the product of millennia of evolution. Muscle, whether of an Olympic athlete or a flying insect, is only around 25% efficient. And most of us function at a much lower level.

If you want to know what a 100% efficient world is like, read *Brave New World*. Real life is messy. We change our minds. We don't even know our own minds. We don't act logically. We start things and then abandon them for something else. We can multitask and anticipate and learn. That flexibility is an effective evolutionary strategy, but it plays havoc with the accountant's bottom line.

In an ideal world every patient would let the practice know when they change their mobile number, their address or their spouse. However many notices we put up in the surgery, it's not going to happen. Nor will every doctor keep every item in the same drawer or remember to use the same computer code for 'heart attack'.

It is a paradox that 'efficiency' became an NHS mantra with Margaret Thatcher, the one prime minister to have a degree in chemistry (second class). She must have known the second law of thermodynamics. Only a system in equilibrium is 100% efficient. Politicians are fighting an impossible battle against entropy. Flu epidemics, natural disasters and health scares ensure that the NHS has to have the flexibility to respond to fluctuations in what is demanded of it, and that means it has to have slack, unless you can conjure doctors, nurses and beds out of thin air. Add patient choice and even more surplus supply is required, unless some patients, like the passengers at the back of the plane, are left with a choice of chicken, chicken or chicken.

The tragedy of 'efficiency savings' is that we could actually save money while improving service to patients, and the professional satisfaction of staff, if we went about it in the right way. Which isn't by demanding a huge budget cut by next December and penalising managers who don't achieve it. The NHS should be asking patients to point out inefficient practices. It should be asking clinical staff, and making the answers public instead of slamming a gagging clause on anyone who points out that things aren't perfect. Sensible patient pathways save everyone time and money. Reducing MRSA infection rates saves a lot of money, but you have to invest in staff to achieve that. Staff are expensive – around 60% of the NHS budget – but good care reduces infection and complication rates, while cheerful, efficient doctors and nurses raise patient morale.

—*NASGP August 2011*

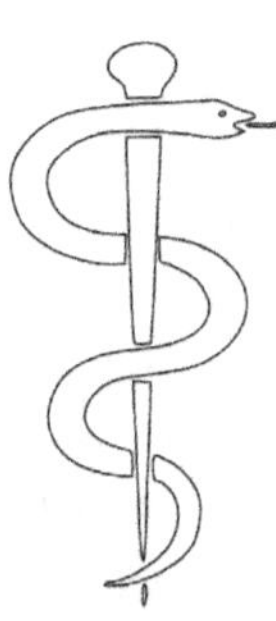

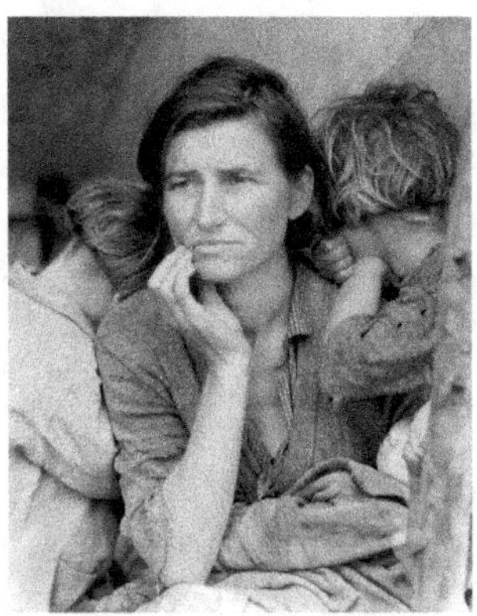

Austerity Kills

I was a medical student. The SHO presented the case, and I asked what the patient did for a living. "He's one of the three million." It was the Thatcher era and unemployment was higher than it had been since the Great Depression. When I came to submit the title for my finals essay, I decided to write about unemployment and health. I was summoned to the Dean's office. I wasn't training to be a social worker, I was reminded. *An Unusual Case of Smith-Bland-Bloggs Syndrome* would be a more appropriate topic.

I stuck to my guns and wrote about the effects of unemployment on health. Clearly, being without work was associated with poor health, and some people were speculating that unemployment was the cause and not the consequence of illness. But they were sociologists, not doctors. Shortly after I qualified, Dr Richard Smith, then the assistant editor of the BMJ, published *Occupationless Health*. Ten articles in the BMJ. The evidence might have been limited but the pain and misery of unemployment were visceral. Since then, there has been a lot of research and I guess that even the more traditional medical schools now recognise that unemployment is bad for your health. Psychological health deteriorates, with increases in suicide and parasuicide rates, especially among young men. Physical health is affected, with slower recovery from minor conditions, more consultations for chronic diseases and more hospital referrals. Poor health affects the whole family, and whole communities as businesses collapse. The pervading threat of joblessness, knowing that the breadwinner's job is precarious, is almost as damaging. And unemployment is bad for us all, as governments save money by cutting public health budgets.

Every unemployment crisis is different. It was the Second

World War that solved the problem of the 1930s. Combatants were promised jobs when they got home, and favourable economic conditions maintained high employment till the 1970s. But by 1979, the Tory election poster read *Labour isn't working*, and by the time I wrote my essay whole industries were disappearing. In the 1990s, statistics appeared to improve, but people were being encouraged to take early retirement, many of the new jobs were part time, and the government was trying to reduce the unemployment figures by encouraging GPs to give the jobless sick notes. Then, as now, governments gained support for cuts in benefits by labelling the out-of-work as scroungers. Health Authorities set up programmes to help the unemployed, but all they could offer were sticking plasters.

The current crisis is different again. We are living longer, with more years to fill and more retirement to support. Women have joined the job market. Everyone expects a standard of material comfort undreamed of in the 1950s. The security of jobs for life has disappeared. Machines take on humans' jobs. Inequality is increasing.

There are now families where no-one has had a paid job for several generations. "Ar ay miss, I'm going to be an artist when I leave school – drawing the dole." So said a 15-year-old I taught in a Liverpool comprehensive school. Those kids weren't interested in learning. All they could foresee was boredom, idleness and purposelessness. No wonder youths turn to drugs to give life some spice, and to gangs for a source of identity and respect.

In capitalist economies a degree of unemployment may be accepted as the inevitable price of economic growth. The USSR guaranteed every citizen a job; in Cuba they still do. But, as Cubans say, "We pretend to work and the government pretends to pay us". Just so: make-work may be better than no work, but it is a poor substitute for a worthwhile job.

Many miners swore that their sons wouldn't go down the pit. But after the pit closures of the 1980s they saw their jobs in a different light. Backbreaking and unpleasant, yes, but a reason to get up in the morning, a pay packet at the end of the week, a useful, and, until the advent of oil, an essential job. And being part of a team, the brotherhood all the stronger because miners shared the arcane hardships of the mines. All are important benefits of even the meanest of employment. Those one-industry communities, the mining towns of the Rhondda Valley, steel towns like Corby, plunged almost overnight from full employment to no employment, and their close-knit societies collapsed. Jobs in construction, which hitherto mopped up the jobless, are in short supply in a recession. The army is cutting back. Even jobs stacking shelves are hard to come as disposable income shrinks.

There are jobs and there are people, but the numbers don't match up, nor do the skills. A sheep shearer who ruins his knee twisting to grab a recalcitrant sheep can't go back to his profession, but neither can he take up a vacancy for an early-Universe cosmologist, even if it is within hobbling distance.

And more and more jobs are being mechanised. Even paying for your toothpaste in Boots. The people who are laid off as a result don't stop existing when their jobs disappear. They still need housing and feeding and health care – more health care than when they were working.

As the cuts introduced to balance the UK budget bite ever deeper, we GPs will see more and more patients whose health is suffering because of unemployment. It feels inevitable. But is it? A new book, *The Body Economic*, by David Stuckler and Sanjay Basu and published this week, shows that debt-burdened countries such as Iceland, or indeed UK in 1945, which decide to maintain health and social spending, not only protect their citizens' health, but recover economically much faster than countries which have opted for austerity. Will our government take note?

I long ago mislaid my finals essay, but Richard Smith's articles are still available on the BMJ website.

—NASGP June 2013

Photo: Migrant mother, Nipomo, California, 1936, by Dorothea Lange

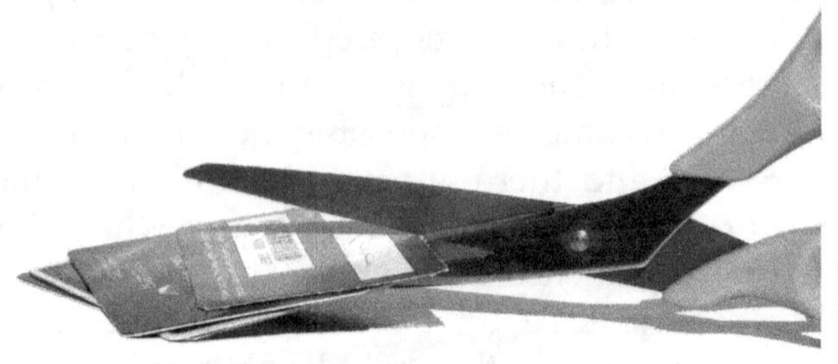

How Would You Cut the NHS Budget?

The NHS budget is going to be cut. Recently the *Today* programme asked for money-saving ideas. Here are some suggestions.

1. Remember that health is a not a commodity and keep the market out of it. Professor Michael Sandel made the argument elegantly in the 2009 Reith lectures.

2. Do not let direct advertising of prescription medication into the UK. And stamp on pharmaceutical advertising aimed at 'disease mongering'.

3. Do not allow doctors a financial stake in businesses which give them an incentive to investigate and hospitalise patients. In his article in the *New Yorker* in June 2009 Atul Gawande illustrates how much this adds to costs and how it actually worsens health outcomes.

4. Educate the public to understand that investigations have a false positive rate, and in a healthy population this is likely to be far higher than the true positive rate. Health care professionals could do with a revision course too. Whoever does the testing, it is the NHS which pays for investigation of these false positives. This is not without risk, and we know that a positive test, even if subsequently negated, permanently undermines people's confidence in their health and increases health-seeking behaviour. Professor Charles Warlow describes his experience of commercial screening in a church in Edinburgh in his recent BMJ article.

5. In my experience of sitting on committees, the smaller the pot of money to be disbursed, the larger and lengthier the meetings called to decide on its fair distribution. Are we reaching the Jarndyce v Jarndyce point at which all the money is spent on making the decision, leaving none for distribution?

6.   Fire the management consultants. I understand that a Primary Care Organisation spent £45,000 on management consultants whose advice led to a saving of £10,000. £35,000 could have financed quite a lot of patient care. Managers are paid high salaries to manage, so how come they have to pay large sums to consultants to tell them what to do? On the *Today* programme, Roy Lilley, terrier of the NHS, opined that many are incompetent. Many GPs would agree.

7.   Put patient benefit at the top of every Primary Care Trust agenda. Anything which directly improves patient care is difficult and seems to take second place to government must-dos and displacement activities like writing 'latex policies'.

8.   Most managers are very remote from patients. I would like to see every manager, including GP practice managers, obliged once a week to walk through a full waiting room and to talk to some of the patients. And to ask themselves every time they launch a policy what difference it will make to the patients they met last week. I recall meetings at a community mental health trust. The board room was near the wards for severely mentally disabled patients, who would wander in during meetings grinding their teeth and grab handfuls of sugar-lumps. They provided a powerful reminder of why we were meeting.

9.   Whatever your view on the regime in Cuba, there can be no doubt that it is a poor country with a first world standard of health. Cuba's expectation of life and infant mortality rates are at least as good as the UK's and better than the USA's – at a fraction of the cost. Yet when planners look around for models for improvement they have a blind spot: the Cuban experience is rarely if ever considered. It should be. Not everything in their health service would work or be acceptable in this country, for social and political reasons, but there may be lessons we can learn, and if we don't look we won't find out.

10.   Educate the public to understand that good health is not a right but a matter of luck, self-help and good sanitation. Doctors and medication play an important, sometimes vital, role, but there is not a pill for every ill, and pills are no substitute for personal effort and attitude. Nor are normal emotional states, such as low mood, shyness and grief, illnesses. And it would help if more people realised that most illnesses are self-limiting and what is needed is time not tablets.

11.   The NHS has a carbon reduction strategy. There are plenty of examples demonstrating that reducing the NHS's huge carbon

footprint can also save money and improve patient care and working lives.

12.   Look hard at prescribing. Medication is a large part of both the NHS budget and its carbon footprint, and much of it is wasted. I recall a patient who came up every month for his pills. When he died a five-year supply was found untouched in his wardrobe. His prescription was a passport to a chat with the dispensers. Many patients who do open the packet take their medication incorrectly, so gain no benefit but risk adverse reactions. Patients accept prescriptions for all sorts of reasons, including over-optimism about the efficacy of pills and a wish not to say no to doctors who are 'doing their best'. And doctors write them for all sorts of reasons with only a tangential relationship with therapeutic efficacy. Doctors need time to establish the sort of relationship with patients so that they are comfortable admitting what they feel about medication and why they don't want to take it.

13.   Walking is good for health, for the environment, and the NHS budget. That applies to staff and patients. Regular exercise improves health and may reduce the need for drug treatment of hypertension, cardiovascular disease, hyperlipidaemia, diabetes, obesity, depression, anxiety, agitation (in both the young and the demented), stress in all its psychological and physical manifestations, many respiratory and rheumatological problems, constipation and no doubt other conditions I haven't thought of.

What are your ideas?

—NASGP August 2009

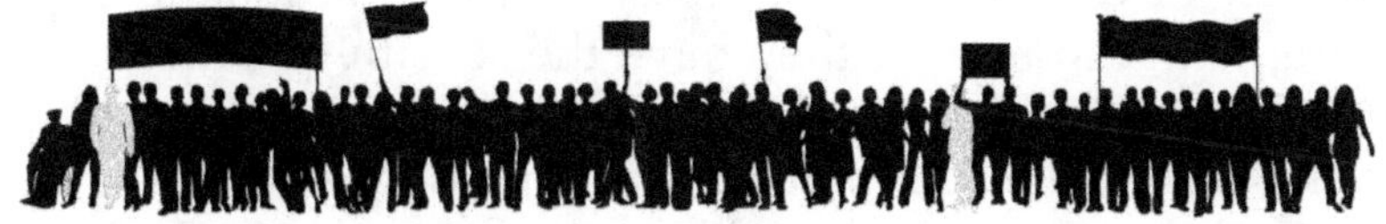

Time to Stand Up and Be Counted

Robert Francis's report on Mid Staffs calls for a change of culture in the NHS. But whose culture is it that needs to change?

Nursing is a tough and poorly paid job. People who choose to become nurses don't expect to find themselves ignoring patients' needs. But when you are rushed off your feet you can't spend time by the bedside to chat to patients. In some hospitals it appears you don't even have time to change soiled sheets. And you can't be kind to a sick patient while you are ticking boxes on your iPad.

Nursing can seem a long way from the image that I absorbed from *Sue Barton, Student Nurse* when I was young. When my elderly mother was admitted to hospital she had a named nurse we were told to speak to about our mother's condition. Only she never seemed to be on duty when we visited and no-one else was prepared to fill the gap. Cheerful caterers put my mum's food on her table, and then cleared it away uneaten. She couldn't see it, and she was too weak to lift a fork. No-one was unkind, but equally no-one seemed to see what was happening, or not happening. Yet there was no glaring deficiency that would put up a red flag to the Trust Board. The Department of Health's statistics would look fine.

The public says bring back matrons. But the root of the problem isn't the culture of nursing. It's too few nurses, too few beds. Beds and nurses cost money. So diabetic patients are on ENT wards, ENT patients on gynaecology wards, any patient on a trolley. At Mid Staffs we have seen the consequences of managing nursing for cost rather than for care.

Doctors seem to have come better out of the Francis report. Though we know that all is not well. A patient asked a GP colleague "Why aren't doctors like Doctor Findlay any more?" He answered "Because patients aren't like Doctor Findlay's patients any more." Social changes have spelt the end of cradle-to-grave continuity of care. But, like nurses, doctors still look after their patients with kindness if they have the sensitivity and the time. These days more hospital doctors introduce themselves to their patients and take the trouble to listen. Evidence-based medicine and case discussions – and legible patient records – make it easier for practice-based GPs to follow up a colleague's patient. GP locums have become expert in the art of creating a therapeutic relationship in 10 minutes.

So whose culture is it that needs to change?

When Tony Blair introduced his reforms of the NHS, I chaired a meeting of local GPs and consultants. A consultant stood up. He and his colleagues, being employees, were increasingly constrained by their employers. You GPs, he said, still have the freedom to plead for your patients. You lose it at your peril. You lose it at your patients' peril. "You must speak out," he urged.

Around the same time I was sitting in the Boardroom of a local Trust at a meeting with the chief executives when the door was pushed open and a man sidled round it. Grunting and grinning and grinding his teeth, he made a dash for the boardroom table, grabbed a handful of sugar-lumps and made his exit. There is something to be said for having a Trust boardroom on the same corridor as a ward for long-stay mentally infirm patients. Too many hospital managers are isolated from patients.

Whose culture needs to change? The government pays lip-service to services for patients, but managers are judged on cost, so the only statistics they see have £ signs in front of them. And whistle-blowing doctors are the messengers bearing bad news. So they are shot. Gagging clauses are now to be banned. But will another way be found to silence those who speak out? It seems that today the NHS is only a no-blame culture if you are at the very top, and kicking the cat goes all the way down the line to the nurses.

And while we're at it, what about the culture of patronising politicians? It isn't motivating to hear an MP saying our performance is mediocre.

What the NHS needs is managing from the bottom up. Why not ask all front-line staff for one thing they could change for the better? It doesn't have to be big: little things mean a lot – and may generate savings too.

Until that culture change happens, it's time for doctors to stand up and shout when patients are suffering. If we don't, who will?

But who's going to listen to a locum? Well, there is strength in numbers. Get together with colleagues. Speak to as many different organisations as you can. Be persistent. And use the media if you have the confidence and the contacts. We are a privileged profession and it is our duty. To the NHS, to patients, to ourselves.

—NASGP April 2013

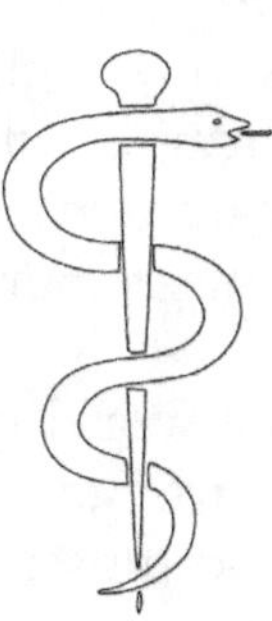

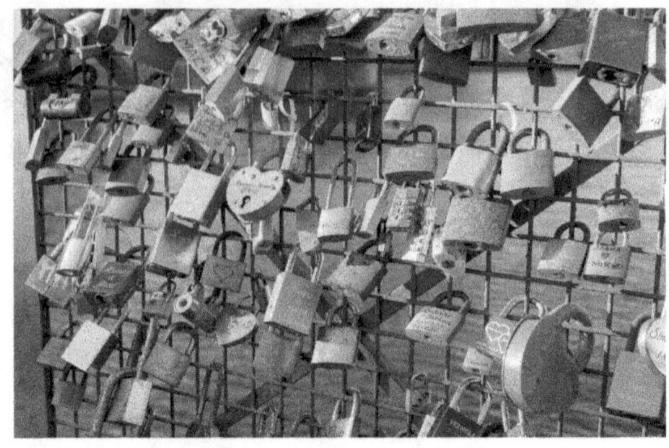

Promises, Promises

It's now a month since the general election, and it didn't turn out as most people expected. But that doesn't mean that the outcome for the NHS will be very different.

How many of the rash promises thrown like sweets at the electorate look likely to be realised? It didn't seem worth reading the manifestos, or even the headline list of undertakings which the parties claimed they were 'locked into'. They all had Houdini clauses to enable the parties to wriggle out of what look like cast-iron commitments. Even carving *An NHS with Time to Care* in stone was never going to guarantee anything.

A few – a very few – themes emerged from the war of words on the NHS.

1.   Labour promised us a world-class health service. Though beloved of managers, it's a strange ambition, since the standard of health care worldwide is nothing to aspire to. And, despite the NHS having fewer of everything (except patients), an independent assessment in 2014 of 11 western health services rated the NHS's performance top in almost every respect.

2.   Jeremy Hunt promised that the Tories would "put GPs at the heart of a revolution in health care". Turns out this means squeezing a seven-day week out of GPs who are already exhausted by five days of unachievable demands. Hunt spent the last parliament fomenting GPs' demoralization, and the last month does not suggest he has realistic plans about rebuilding what he has done so much to damage.

3.   Everyone promised that patients will get an appointment today/at any time of day/night/every day of the year/NOW. It's unrealistic. Oh, so it's an aspiration? Just as well: it will take years

to train the extra staff. Oh, and the promises are for patients who 'need' an appointment? Who will determine a patient's 'need'? In the consumer-oriented society that successive governments have fostered, that's the consumer's choice, isn't it?

4.   Shorter waiting times for secondary care. We would all like that. But, again, where will the doctors come from, and does the budget, if one exists, include not just their salaries, but those of ancillary staff, equipment and additional buildings required?

5.   Money. There was a hot bidding war. It may have sounded like megabucks, but even the highest bid would barely meet the current shortfall. Eighty percent of acute trusts have overspent their budgets. Are they *all* inefficient and profligate? Or is it simply impossible to provide a decent standard of care with the money they have been allocated? Private providers like Serco think so; they have opted out and left it to the public purse to take over.

6.   Three percent efficiency savings year on year – till the budget approaches zero? There will always be inefficiencies but the profits demanded by private providers may cost more. And some 'inefficiencies' provide essential flexibility. To an accountant, unoccupied beds in July is overprovision, but having too few beds in January is inefficient and costs lives.

Many things important to those who work in the NHS and to patients were not addressed in the election sound bites.

1.   A lot was – is – said about getting patients into hospital. Little is said about getting them out again. There are bottlenecks all through the system, starting with ambulances queuing outside hospitals waiting for a bed/trolley/board to become free. But the ultimate rate-limiting step is discharge. Patients used to stay in hospital for 10 days after routine surgery. Now that stays are down to 48 hours, patients are more vulnerable. And they are likely to be older, so less likely to have someone at home who can care for them as they convalesce. Amalgamating health and social care doesn't solve the problem if there is no money to provide home care.

2.   Flexibility. Yes. But only where it's appropriate. Farming out an elderly man with epistaxis to the orthopaedic ward, or even to a gynae side ward, is monumentally inefficient. And dangerous. ENT nurses know about managing potentially lethal nosebleeds. Orthopaedic nurses don't.

3.   False economies. When Monitor is on your back about your overspend, the easiest cut is salaries. But it costs, even in the short run. Experienced staff provide better value for money than

younger, cheaper replacements. Slash your established workforce to dangerous levels and you have to plug the gaps. But agency staff, however able they are, don't have local experience and the loyalties which make an effective team. They are very expensive. As the government is realising. But it looks as if it is too late to rebuild a stable, valued, efficient workforce. The staff have left the NHS and it will take years to retrain replacements.

4.   How long before governments realise that care in the community doesn't necessarily save money? Hospitals have economy of scale. Paring down community costs by not paying staff for travel time between patients is immoral.

5.   Technology, yes: SMS, down-the-line results. But despite huge investments in IT, too many hospital consultations are frustrated because the doctor doesn't have the patient's notes. Why not turn the problem around and put all the notes on a patient-help smart card? Probably fewer records would be lost than currently go missing in hospitals. And every health care professional could add their notes, every prescriber could check a patient's history and medication and add their new drug safely to the list.

6.   Elastoplast is cheap but no treatment for serious problems. Politicians think short term, NHS staff have a longer view. Leave the bright ideas to them.

Underlying all the words is the assumption that money, allocating more or squeezing more out of each £, can enable the NHS to make us live for ever. So we don't die of heart disease, or cancer, or dementia. The rhetoric misses the point, that the major determinant of health is your social condition. People living in nice houses and earning decent incomes live years longer than those who live a mile away on meagre benefits in dilapidated housing. It's the survival of the richest. But that is a nettle no political party hoping to form a government will grasp.

Despite the onslaughts, the NHS is kept going by enthusiastic and dedicated, if increasingly weary, staff. And they have lots of ideas. Look at the submissions for the 2015 BMJ Awards and be inspired.

—NASGP June 2015

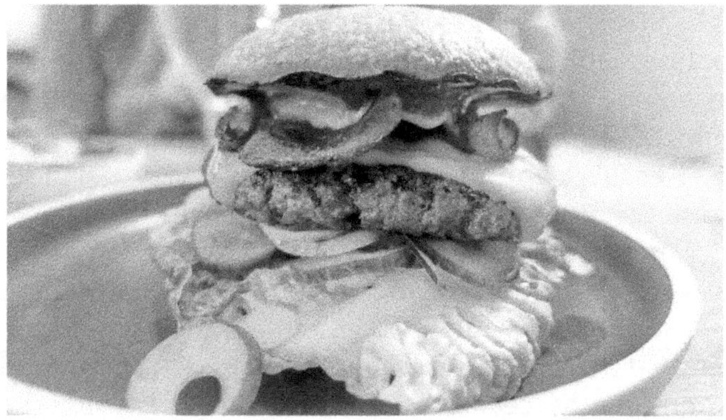

Should GPs Take On the Takeaways?

You don't need scales and height-weight charts to realise that people are fatter than they used to be. It's clear that obesity is already damaging patients, and that in years to come it will take a huge toll on the nation's health.

As GPs we have always tackled our patients' obesity. Now we are going to be commissioning. What obesity services should we commission?

Homo sapiens evolved to exploit any opportunity to eat. Humans are not programmed to exercise restraint. But now food is abundant, our lives don't demand physical exertion, and restraint is out of fashion. So is drudgery. The food industry has responded to provide immediate gratification and foster a culture of grazing and snacking at all hours – and not on raw carrots.

It's not just what we eat outside the home. Apparently 75% of the nation's diet is now processed food, carefully formulated to increase the desire for more . . . and more . . . and more. It slips straight down so it doesn't stimulate satiety, so we buy super-sized portions, bolstered with salt and sugar to increase both customers' satisfaction and companies' profits. And now around 60% of the population are overweight.

What can be done? There is no putting back the clock – mother in a pinny serving up a home-cooked roast meat and two veg to husband and two children, forks at the ready at the family dining table. Those days are gone. The British have given up cooking. Thirty years ago, people on a budget stewed root vegetables with the extremities of quadrupeds. But these days, economic stringency isn't driving people back to the kitchen stove. Rather, they choose cheaper pizzas.

It has been suggested that GPs should use every consultation to advise patients about obesity. It would certainly sour relationships if patients knew that consulting over a sore toe would include a nag about their diet, but it wouldn't do much for the obesity problem. Kernels of information have to fall on fertile ground. If everyone behaved logically no-one under the age of 60 would smoke. Even doctors seek comfort in chocolate.

Sensitively given, information *is* important. Most people still have a sense of what is good for them, or they wouldn't tell the practice nurse that they eat tons of fresh greens when in fact they buy all their food at Iceland. So advice which seems to fall on deaf ears may bear fruit (and veg) later on. Food labelling is useful, but reading labels takes time and literacy and commitment. How many people bother, unless they are worried the contents might make them seriously ill? Similarly, only the motivated will stick with a weight management programme, and only if it works. A recent BMJ editorial reported that NHS services have a lot to learn from Weight Watchers about the value of regular group sessions, intensive support and incentives.

If we can't change people, perhaps we can change environmental factors which influence food choices. Kids don't like queuing for school dinners because it cuts into playtime. As well as banning fast-food vans, some enterprising councils provide vans which serve up food from the school canteen so that pupils can grab a fast but healthy lunch.

There is also what is now called nudging – changing social norms. It worked with drink-driving. Nudging the British public into choosing healthier foods is a bigger challenge, but serving burgers with salads instead of chips would be a start. More exercise would also help. Selling off playing fields was a nudge in the wrong direction.

But this is tinkering. We have to tackle processed food. Not easy. We are up against an industry that has the power to get pizza reclassified at a vegetable. Yes, the food industry pressured the US authorities to take this Alice in Wonderland decision! And we are up against the *Daily Mail*, ever poised to rage against the nanny state – which gives consumers a cop-out.

"Make the healthy choice the easy choice", says WHO. It can be done. Regulation plays a part – restricting advertising to children and reducing trans fats in processed food. It has been suggested that increasing the price of sugar would both please farmers and encourage manufacturers to cut down the sugar in their products or switch to cheaper, healthier sweeteners. The tax system could be used to make the healthy choice the cheap choice. Financial incentives could enable corner shops to offer fresher, healthier food.

Surprisingly, it appears that voluntary agreements can work. Over some years, several big manufacturers have reduced the salt content of foods, so slowly that consumers don't notice. Such products aren't advertised as 'low salt'. That would kill sales. But they are always changing unobtrusively, and this change has lasting health benefits.

What about the 25% of food eaten outside the home? It's a challenge; takeaways have very low margins and customers want to know the price, not the fat content of their fish and chips. But in Belfast, following workshops in Cantonese and a Masterchef competition, 68% of Chinese takeaways improved their food. Lincoln has a similar project with Indian takeaways. And even something as simple as providing salt shakers with five holes instead of seventeen can make a difference.

So what can we do, as clinicians and commissioners? Here are some suggestions.

1.   Continue to inform and remind patients, sensitively, about the risks of obesity and how to eat healthily.

2.   Know about effective dietary advice, support groups and weight loss programmes in our area.

3.   Set up partnerships with councils and other local organisations to improve the availability of healthy food. Spread information about it.

4.   Then doctors can offer real-world advice. We can direct patients to the healthiest pizzas, tandooris, Chinese takeaways. And after a long evening surgery, we might follow our own advice.

—*NASGP February 2012*

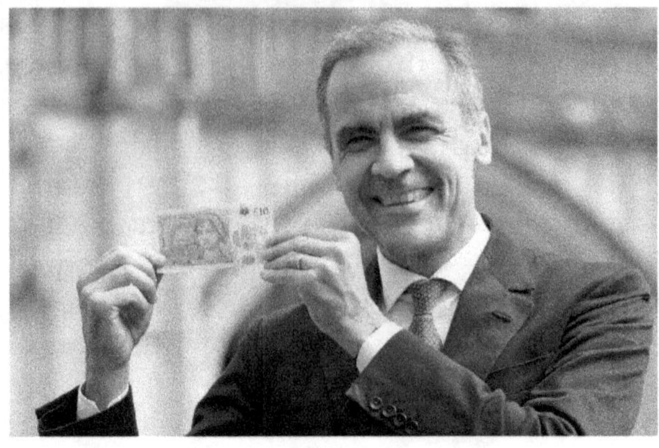

Are You in It for the Money?

People try lots of ways to get other people to work harder: bonuses, performance-related pay, incentive schemes, targets, QOF, profit shares, fee for service, commission, piece work, payment by results, stock options . . . all are carrots to extract more work from staff. But how effective are they?

The evidence is, not very. As I found out for myself.

Twenty years ago I was a partner in a practice which had a staff bonus system. I was commissioned to write an article for a general practice magazine. They expected me to say how motivating it was for staff to share in the practice's profits. I described how we were abandoning it because it had proved so demotivating.

A difficult year had put strains on the team and on the practice finances. Everyone deserved a bonus but there wasn't any money. "Yes, we know," they said, "but where is my bonus?" They had come to take the share-out for granted. Perhaps they had already spent it.

Even in a good year distributing the pot was an uncomfortable process. Were we rewarding effort or achievement? How do you rate a valuable member of staff who has underperformed this year because she has been nursing her sick mother versus the loyal employee who tries her best, but whose best is not in all honesty much good? How to handle the delicate problem that a partner's daughter works in the practice and her father values her contribution much more highly then his partners do? And the less there is in the pot, the more agonising it is deciding how to share it out.

How else can you show staff that they are appreciated? A bottle of booze at Christmas? No good for non-drinkers. Knick-knacks?

Embarrassing to find them recycled at the local bring-and-buy. A weekend in Paris (after a very good year)? Some people don't want to go to Paris, others don't want to go without their spouses, the youngest partner drinks too much and behaves inappropriately – very inappropriately – at the celebratory dinner. And it rains. Bonding? No.

I have discovered that there is whole industry trying to design incentives that provide maximum motivation with minimum opportunity for abuse. All such schemes involve changing the goal posts frequently to keep staff on their toes, but none is effective in the long term; in fact the reverse. In the real world, you can't eliminate the possibilities for gaming, and gaming is what humans do. If there is a bounty on rats' tails, people will breed rats.

But those in charge continue to believe in financial incentives. Successive governments have attempted to squeeze more out of general practice. They have tried to combine the carrot of better pay with the reward of better care of patients, but there seems to be little evidence that patients are healthier as a result. If a higher level of QOF payment can be reached by eliminating more patients from the denominator, few practices will resist the temptation to search their list for exceptions to report. They may then reach the target, but it won't be a joyful experience.

Whatever they say, governments and big organisations like top-down solutions. Providing extrinsic rewards enables them to tick their boxes. And if million-pound bonuses are necessary to reward bankers for doing their job, they feel that a few crumbs will screw more productivity – as defined by them – out of the NHS's huge workforce. But few people work in the NHS solely for the money. They value the opportunity to exercise their skills. They value teamwork. They value solving problems. They value the feeling that they are helping people.

Teams will strive to meet goals they have set for themselves. In the past many GPs felt that, however desirable it might be to check every patients' blood pressure, it was unrealistic. In 1974 Dr Julian Tudor Hart's Welsh mining town practice set itself a challenge: to measure the blood pressure of every patient in the practice. They showed that it could be done, and that patients whose hypertension was identified and managed lived longer.

Being part of a team with a shared purpose is a big motivator. Soldiers will lay their down their lives for their mates. On the front line of the NHS, your contribution doesn't have to be heroic. For months everyone has seen the stained chair in the waiting room that no patient ever wants to sit on. If you have the courage to take it away, your colleagues cheer. And the best thing the boss can give is not monetary reward but acknowledgement. Although the US government has only one vice-president, American companies have platoons of them. Why? Because recognition is an effective cheap way of fostering motivation. It doesn't have to be a title; in the NHS, a smile and a word of appreciation go a long way, but they are often forgotten.

NHS staff have been flocking to make *Change Day* pledges. It's exhilarating to see your pledge earning dozens of 'likes'. Wherever you are, through the web and social media you can feel part of something big.

I don't know how many of the half a million *Change Day* pledges come from GP locums, but a good few locums will have made New Year resolutions. Good-enough practice may be good enough to make a capable doctor, but exercising your own imagination and meeting your own challenges is what professional satisfaction is all about.

—NASGP April 2014

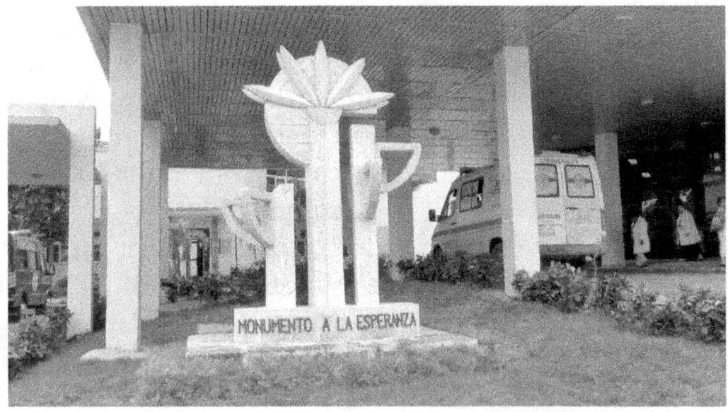

The Doctor Factory

After the Cuban Revolution, Fidel Castro made health and education a priority. In 1959 he said "I invite everyone who has the vocation to study medicine". Last year, as well as the 4,800 students from 70 other countries who trained on full scholarships from the Cuban government, 5,600 native Cuban doctors graduated. Britain produces around 8,000 new doctors every year. The population of Cuba is one-sixth of ours, so the equivalent figure in Britain would be over 33,000.

What do they do with them all? Many work abroad; they are Cuba's diplomatic weapon.

In 1960 Castro sent 56 health workers to Algeria on a 14-month assignment. Since then the number of Cuban doctors working overseas has multiplied, and an increasing number of medical students qualify each year to feed the demand. Currently there are around 20,000 Cuban doctors working overseas on long-term projects in 100 countries, from Venezuela to Vanuatu. Additionally Cuba sends teams to every natural disaster. Well, nearly every natural disaster: President Bush declined Castro's offer of help after Hurricane Katrina.

There are other objectors. When Brazil's president Dilma Rousseff responded to street protests over dire public services by hiring 4,500 Cuban doctors, local medics criticised their standard of care and tried to discredit their qualifications – unsuccessfully. It's true that it is difficult to assess their outcomes, but independent evidence from Honduras shows that maternal and infant mortality fell dramatically in areas where Cubans had been working. And the complication rate of Cuba's *Operación Milagro* cataract programme appears to be acceptable.

Cuban doctors are sent to remote areas and no-go inner city *barrios*, where millions of poor people have never seen a doctor because local medics will not work there. Maybe these professionals will be shamed into changing their attitudes by seeing Cuban doctors, many of them from poor backgrounds, many of them black, serving poor communities.

Cubans doctors are sometimes suspected of being covert intelligence agents, though the opportunities must be limited for doctors working in, say, Tuvalu, or for the two who found themselves trapped in Karbala during the Iran-Iraq war and operated day and night for months while the bombs fell.

Tellingly, many countries, international organisations and NGOs have sufficient confidence in Cuba's health programmes to use them as a funnel for aid money. Norway contributed $2 million for Cuba's emergency work in Haiti. Pan American Health Organization, which is WHO's American arm, supports Cuba's health education work in Latin America. Eighty-five NGOs worldwide have subsidised Cuba's Comprehensive Health Programs in Africa.

The doctors are the front line of Cuba's medical diplomacy. They are trained with a service ethic, and they know that someday they will be called upon to serve. It's also an adventure and a chance to travel, an opportunity unavailable to most Cubans. They earn more while they are overseas, and they're allowed to send home the sort of consumer goods it's hard to get in Cuba.

And they may defect. It seems unlikely that many teenagers choose to study medicine because it might offer opportunities to escape, but some doctors do jump ship while they are abroad. It's impossible to determine how many: probably more than the Cubans admit to but less than the US government, which has in the past offered inducements, hoped. And I don't know the truth about confiscation of passports and surveillance by 'minders'.

There are personal costs. It seems you can refuse to go if you have a good reason, but pressure will be applied on you to go next time. And it is hard on families. As a woman who spent five years as a single parent while her ophthalmologist husband worked in Venezuela said to me, "It's a sacrifice".

For the state of Cuba doctors are an export. Disaster relief apart, countries pay the Cuban government for the doctors: 28% of Cuba's export earnings come from selling medical services. Venezuela pays in oil which has kept Cuba going for the past fifteen years. Poor countries are charged less than wealthier ones.

Some Cubans grumble when waiting times lengthen because doctors have gone overseas, but most are proud of what their country is doing. The benefits aren't just financial. Cuba has won the admiration and support of nations around the world. Only the USA, Israel and Palau now support the US economic blockade of Cuba. Brazil and Qatar are investing in big projects in Cuba and other countries are signing bilateral agreements. Symbolic capital is converting into material capital. The prestige will stand Cuba in good stead.

What are the ethics of Cuba's medical diplomacy? Cubans don't have much choice about serving overseas. They know that is how they will repay their government for funding their training, just as UK students have to pay back the loan which financed their training. Are their doctors providing international aid and development, or are they an arm of the diplomatic corps, or a quasi-military service? Perhaps a bit of all three. They provide deprived populations with essential medical services. They train local people. They are an advertisement for their country.

How does a nation win hearts and minds? Western military efforts in Afghanistan seem to have failed miserably and the British are withdrawing from Helmand. Drones create enemies. Doctors win friends.

—NASGP February 2014

Photo: Hospital in Havana

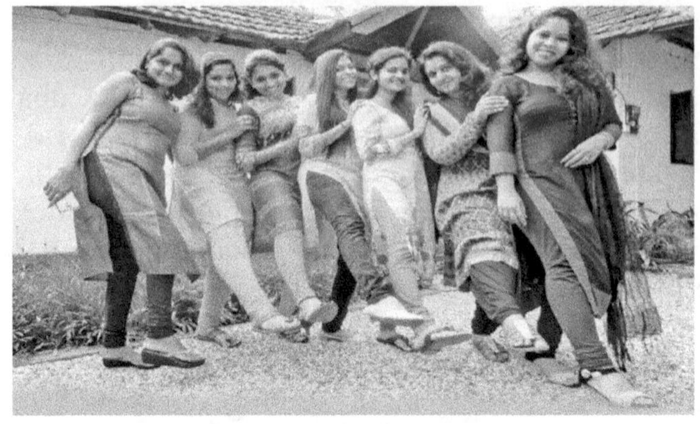

Leggislating Change

What had changed in the 15 years since I was last in India? I would never have guessed: leggings. Women everywhere were wearing them.

And Prime minister Narendra Modi had just announced demonetisation, a bold measure to tackle corruption. From midnight on 8th November 2016 the banknotes which comprised 85% of India's currency were no longer legal tender. The result was economic chaos.

Why do some innovations catch on when others are disastrous? An Indian journalist described demonetisation as "a bad idea, badly executed on the basis of some half-baked notions." Many have said the same about reorganisations of the NHS. The health service is no stranger to top-down imposition of change.

Governments' horizons are usually short-term. The possible unintended consequences of their policies are an inconvenient truth which is given scant consideration; implementation is someone else's problem.

Only one person knew in advance about Modi's demonetisation plan – the governor of the Reserve Bank of India, who had to arrange printing of new bank notes. It's true that the NHS – usually – goes through a process of consultation, if a brick through the window constitutes listening to the people who actually provide and use the health service.

Following demonetisation there weren't nearly enough banknotes to go round so millions of Indians queued every day, waiting to change their now-useless savings. Businesses went bust, people could not buy or sell. They had no money for food and crops rotted in the fields.

Reorganisations of the NHS can quickly demonstrate flaws in new policies – think of Andrew Lansley's disastrous 2012 Health and Social Care Act. But front-line staff still have to carry on. Bank staff in India faced millions of desperate people. NHS clinicians do their best to keep the health service going for patients while getting their heads round the new demands and new structures.

When the Department of Health is criticised in the press and in parliament, GPs are convenient fall-guys. It is not the failure of primary care to embrace seven-day services that is causing the nationwide crisis in A&E, but by the time that point was made, the popular press had ensured that every prejudice against GPs had been reinforced.

Unless they make a big effort to stay in touch, the decision-makers in governments and large organisations are insulated from the day-to-day reality of the people they are supposed to serve. By the time a policy has filtered down through layers of management, what may have seemed like a surgical strike has turned into something resembling carpet bombing.

Unfortunately the pressure is on general practices to form bigger organisations. Whatever the potential gains, as the lines of communications are lengthened the opportunity for big mistakes which are difficult to unpick will increase.

Effective change usually happens from the bottom up. Checking capillary refill time wasn't mentioned when I trained and it seems that it only entered the literature 10 years ago. I don't suppose many high-level managers know what it means. Yet now it is a test every GP uses. It costs nothing, is easy for both the doctor and the patient, and it gives useful information. So it caught on quickly. As did pulse oximeters. They were first widely used by US anaesthetists in the 1980s, then hospital practitioners picked up on them. They are easy and quick to use and the information they provide is cheap at the price and helps decision-making. Now few GPs would want to be without one.

Endomysial antibody and faecal calprotectin tests have both proved their usefulness, as has guidance on sepsis, and the vast majority of GPs will be familiar with them. When a few innovators introduced self-referral to physiotherapists, physio services were not overwhelmed. GPs' time was saved, patients were happy with direct and quick access and outcomes improved. Now self-referral is the norm and other services are taking it up. The idea wasn't handed down from above; it caught on because people who tried it found that it was effective. Similarly one-stop clinics and one-stop assessment centres have worked to everyone's advantage and the models have been copied and adapted for use in different places and circumstances.

What gets the ball rolling? Rarely governments; they are busy devising carrots and sticks to urge forward their latest must-dos. Good ideas spread like dandelions in a field. Word of mouth propelled Dr Henry Heimlich's manoeuvre into everyday usage and significantly reduced the death toll from choking. Articles in the press, meetings, websites can be catalysts of change. And locums. Unlike partners, they see a lot of practices in action, and their employers are recognising that a locum's skills and experience are a useful resource. Practice B has a problem. A locum can tell them how practice A found a neat way of solving the problem. Partners who learned their trade using paper notes can ask a young IT-savvy locum how things could be done more easily. And then practices pass on the advice.

Back to leggings. Nobody in the government demanded that Indian women wear leggings. In fact, politicians probably see them as a threat to tradition. But women found them cheap and practical, and now leggings are available everywhere, in bazaars, on pavement stalls, online. A change that comes from the ground up.

—*NASGP February 2017*

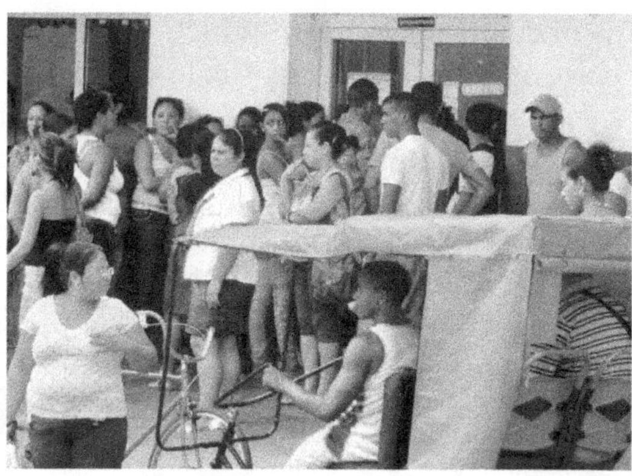

"No Es Fácil"

Few things in Cuba are easy. Most countries faced with what Cuba has lived with for more than half a century would be failed states. Cuba keeps going, with hardship and sacrifice, but a shared vision.

The reputation of Cuba's health service – providing rich-country outcomes on a poor-country budget – attracts interest from politically aware medical students. But arranging an elective there, well, *no es fácil*. Fidel Castro's *Escuela Latinoamericana de Medicina* provides medical training for poor students from other countries, but few people in Cuba's health service are aware that medical training worldwide often includes an elective. Only the occasional foreign student managed to penetrate the indifference, the bureaucracy, the lack of information and the limitations of Cuba's IT to arrange an elective.

I was fortunate to meet a Cuban doctor with the imagination to think outside the restrictive Cuban box. He had welcomed one such applicant. We discussed the practicalities of an elective programme, and in 2010 I started Cuba Medical Link, a UK registered charity with a website to help students arrange electives in Cuba. Eight years, 400 students from 20 countries later, I have closed this programme.

No es fácil, an elective in Cuba. Foreign students are in Cuba on Cuba's terms. They pay substantial fees for their tuition. They have to speak Spanish. They learn alongside Cuban medical students, they live as paying guests with Cuban families. Being Cuban *no es fácil*, and students gain an insight into the difficulties of everyday life under the USA's economic blockade. They acquire a first-hand experience of the Cuban health system and of the social sacrifices and restrictions of political freedom which underpin it.

Once they have surmounted the hurdles of registering in Cuba and donned a *bata blanca* (white coat) elective students enter a world of shared knowledge of the human body and its infirmities. Cuban doctors are generally welcoming and keen to teach. But practising in Cuba *no es fácil.* Buildings may be in need of basic repairs, and doctors may have only a thin, shabby towel to dry their hands. But the commitment to patients is the same. Cuban ingenuity keeps antiquated CT scanners working 24/7 and every stroke patient is scanned in A&E – an objective few British hospitals achieve.

Back home, students probably don't think much about the patient's diagnosis till they have the results of a battery of investigations. Cuban students have to learn to make a diagnosis without technology, and elective students have to try to do the same. As one British student said, "I felt like an amateur compared to their seemingly vast clinical skills!"

Some differences can be startling. Interactions with patients can sometimes be uncomfortably brusque. And in a country in which people live in each others' pockets, confidentiality isn't a consideration. It can be a shock to find two doctors consulting in the same small room and all available space crammed with patients' relatives and friends, nurses, medical students and even the next patient who has wandered in through the open door.

In many countries preventative health care is given only lip service, or responsibility is devolved to public health departments. Visiting students see how in Cuba it is everyone's responsibility, and they make the connection with Cuba's impressive health statistics. They may even take part: a Japanese student was proud to give a talk about reducing their risk of heart disease to a group of *abuelos* (elderly) at their exercise class. As another student observed "The primary care doctor in Cuba is part shaman, part confessor and this demonstrates both their medical and social roles and how it is difficult, and probably inappropriate, to try to see one without the other."

Students go to the beach, play football, go dancing with their fellow Cuban students. Cuban doctors teach them to interpret X-rays and to make a *mojito,* and most welcome the opportunity to find out how medicine is practiced in the students' home country. Students put the world to rights and go to meditation classes with their Cuban *casa* hosts.

For one student his elective fulfilled a childhood ambition.

When he was 14 his mother agreed to buy him a Che Guevara T-shirt on condition that he read Che's biography, and he became fascinated by Cuba.

For Cubans the students open a window on a different world. The Indian parents of one British student came to visit during her elective. "We had a big dinner with the two families which was a mixture of Cuban, English and Indian food with a healthy amount of Cuban rum afterwards. Our hostess is fascinated by Indian culture but will probably never see the real India. I like to think in some way our visit allowed her and her family to understand a little more about other cultures as much as it helped us to do so."

Almost every student report was positive; for some it was a life-changing experience. But the barriers to setting up and running a functional programme were substantial and the process was exhausting.

Cuban medical school authorities were full of goodwill, but they face huge obstacles. They may share a computer with several colleagues, it may work erratically, and probably struggles to download a one-page document. Most Cubans have no experience of the way other countries do things, and some found it hard to understand the need to keep students informed. Some applications sat in piles in an office while the students' deadline for confirming their electives expired. One Cuban official was frustrated that forms from medical schools around the world aren't all the same, as forms are in Cuba.

Only one independent-minded official answered emails promptly, didn't ignore sensitive questions, and understood that students have to change their plans if they fail their exams or break a leg.

And he did his best to be flexible. Cubans may be agile and inventive on the dance floor, but these are not qualities which get you very far up the ladder in a totalitarian state. And Cuba is very suspicious of foreign intervention – with reason. So the programme began, like most start-ups, under the radar. It took some years to get an appointment with someone in MINSAP – the Ministry of Health. Though official recognition didn't make a lot of difference.

They do things differently in Cuba. In one centre, the woman responsible for dealing with students' electives went on holiday for three weeks and no-one looked at her emails, or, apparently, knew she was away. Without notice, the government closed the bank account through which students paid their fees, throwing a score of electives into doubt. It took time before alternative arrangements were made. At one point some remote bureaucratic action abruptly doubled tuition fees and imposed an impossible, expensive and Kafkaesque system of accrediting documents. The programme was on the edge of collapse until we achieved a reprieve.

Administration was onerous and unremunerated. It took time to sift from the five hundred or so enquiries I received each year the 40 or 50 students with a genuine interest, adequate Spanish and money to pay the fees. And sorting out the bureaucratic problems they encountered in dealing with Cuba never got easier.

Over the years I sought a sustainable future for the programme. *No era fácil*. In fact, *imposible*. Medical schools were interested, but only for their own students. The government's Department for International Trade accompanies the RCGP on trips to China, but isn't interested in a country with very limited investment opportunities. No charity was interested in sponsorship. No business, NGO, Global Health department, student elective organisation, wanted to take on unremunerated work. The logical place for the administration is Cuba, but that clearly is not feasible. I couldn't carry on, so had no option but to close the programme.

I am puzzled and disappointed that so few students – only 10% – gave me any feedback. Not even clicking 'reply' to my welcome home email to offer one tip for future students. Those that did send reports gave vivid pictures of the reality of Cuba's health service, something no tourist or visiting official ever sees. I just hope that all the students take into their careers some of the lessons they learnt in Cuba.

Around 400 students had an unforgettable experience, forged friendships, and had their horizons broadened and their assumptions tested. Where else can you get a political education while enjoying sun, sand and salsa?

—NASGP December 2017

Photo: Queuing in Santiago de Cuba

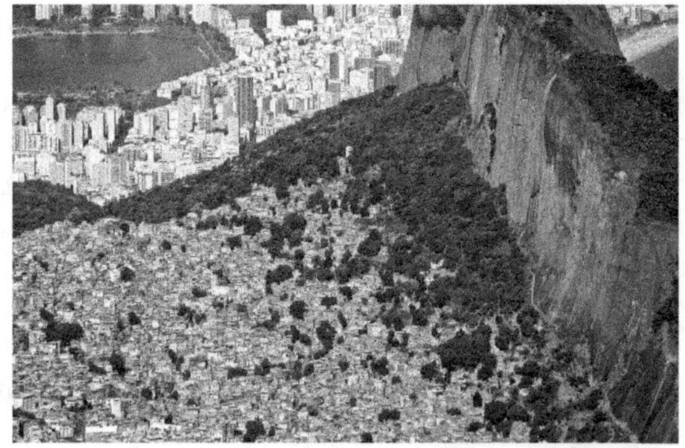

Why No Man Is an Island

If you plot a graph of the wealth of nations against the health of their citizens, it is clear that, up to a point, the more you spend the better the health outcomes. But if you then analyse the health of the rich countries that cluster at the top of the graph, where extra spending has ceased to buy significant gains in health, something very interesting emerges. The more equal the society, the better the health of its citizens. And not just their health: on a wide range of social measurements equal societies score better. In contrast, societies where a small percentage of people hold most of the wealth, everyone, rich or poor, is less healthy, less comfortable and less fulfilled. In the UK, now one of the least equal countries, we have never been so anxious about being happy.

The Spirit Level, written by two British epidemiologists, examines the phenomenon in detail, plotting physical and mental health, teenage pregnancy rates, children's educational performance, community violence and levels of trust against the level of inequality in 23 countries of the rich world, and also against the level of inequality in the states of the USA. In almost every case, the problems are worse, often much worse, in unequal societies. There is no evidence that this is due to confounding factors: inequality appears to be at the root of many of the social ills which occupy news headlines.

Intuitively, the idea seems right. Gang warfare and the demand for respect which fuels it are responses to inequality. The rich may try to isolate themselves in gated communities, but electronic barriers, security guards and razor wire cannot entirely eliminate the fear and anxiety which must gnaw away at their enjoyment and their health. The costs of managing the problems of inequality suck money from the services which should be promoting equality: responding to the democratically expressed wish of its citizens to control antisocial behaviour, the government of California now spends more on prisons than on education.

The society most people dream of living in is an equal one – everyone in the village drinking in the same pub and sharing the pleasures of the summer fete. Though humans quarrel over resources, we also co-operate, and the pleasure we get from group activities is demonstrated way beyond the football field and the orchestra. There is a balance between our hierarchical and our co-operative natures.

The ideas in *The Spirit Level* are not new. I first came across them in a BMJ editorial in 1996, It was a 'eureka moment', and I still have on file the series of articles under the title *Socioeconomic Determinants of Health*, edited by *Spirit Level* author Richard Wilkinson, which followed. And in 2008, the report by Michael Marmot, chair of the WHO commission on social determinants in health, declared "Social injustice is killing people on a grand scale".

So, since equality is good for us all, what can be done to promote it? Ironically, war fosters equality. Faced with an external threat, we all pull together. But there are other ways of generating equal societies, and it doesn't matter how the equality is achieved. Both Japan and Sweden score well on equality. In Japan, there is a narrow range of incomes, while Sweden has a much wider disparity between incomes but a progressive taxation system which redistributes wealth. Even inside the USA the same is found: New Hampshire and Vermont both score highly on equality, but in New Hampshire income is evenly distributed while in Vermont it is redistributed through tax.

"There is no such thing as society: there are individual men and women, and there are families," said Margaret Thatcher, setting the tone which accompanied the growth of inequality in this country. But in reality we are all in the same boat, and on the same planet, and not just our happiness but our survival depend on us pulling together. How can we persuade our politicians and those who soar in the financial stratosphere earning hundreds of times more than most of the rest of us, that equality is good for all of us, poor or rich? Put another way, how can we start to reaccumulate the social capital that we have thrown away over the past twenty years?

Well, there is an election coming up. The government has

responded to economic collapse by trying everything it can think of to stimulate economic growth. The opposition is pursuing the same solution. But where is the evidence that economic growth is going to mend our 'broken society'? There seems to be no voice speaking out for using the collapse to forge a different strategy. No-one is pointing out to the wealthy that it is in their interest, not just that of the poor, to review the way companies are run and the level of rewards of those who currently command stratospheric incomes. The easy way for a government to be seen to be doing something is to slap on a sticking plaster, and that is what most politicians are proposing. But these problems are gaping wounds, and exhortations to eat green vegetables, lectures on the dangers of obesity and posters about knife crime don't change society. So when the election candidates come knocking on your door, ask them what they plan to do for equality. And check the website of *The Equality Trust* to see what you can do.

📖 ***The Spirit Level*** *Richard Wilkinson and Kate Pickett, 2009*

—NASGP April 2010

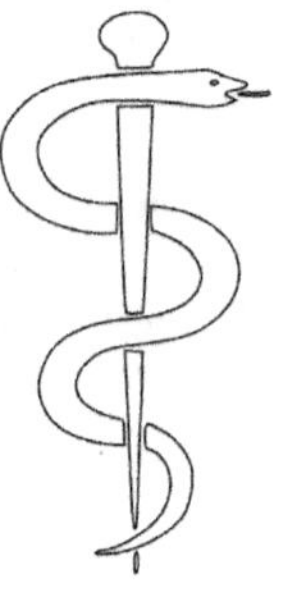

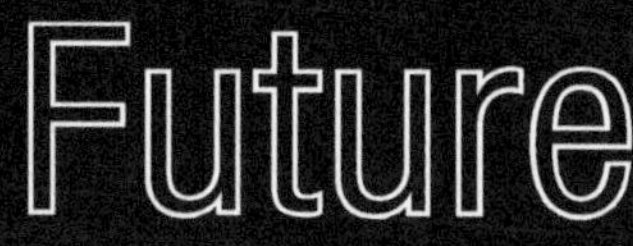

Future

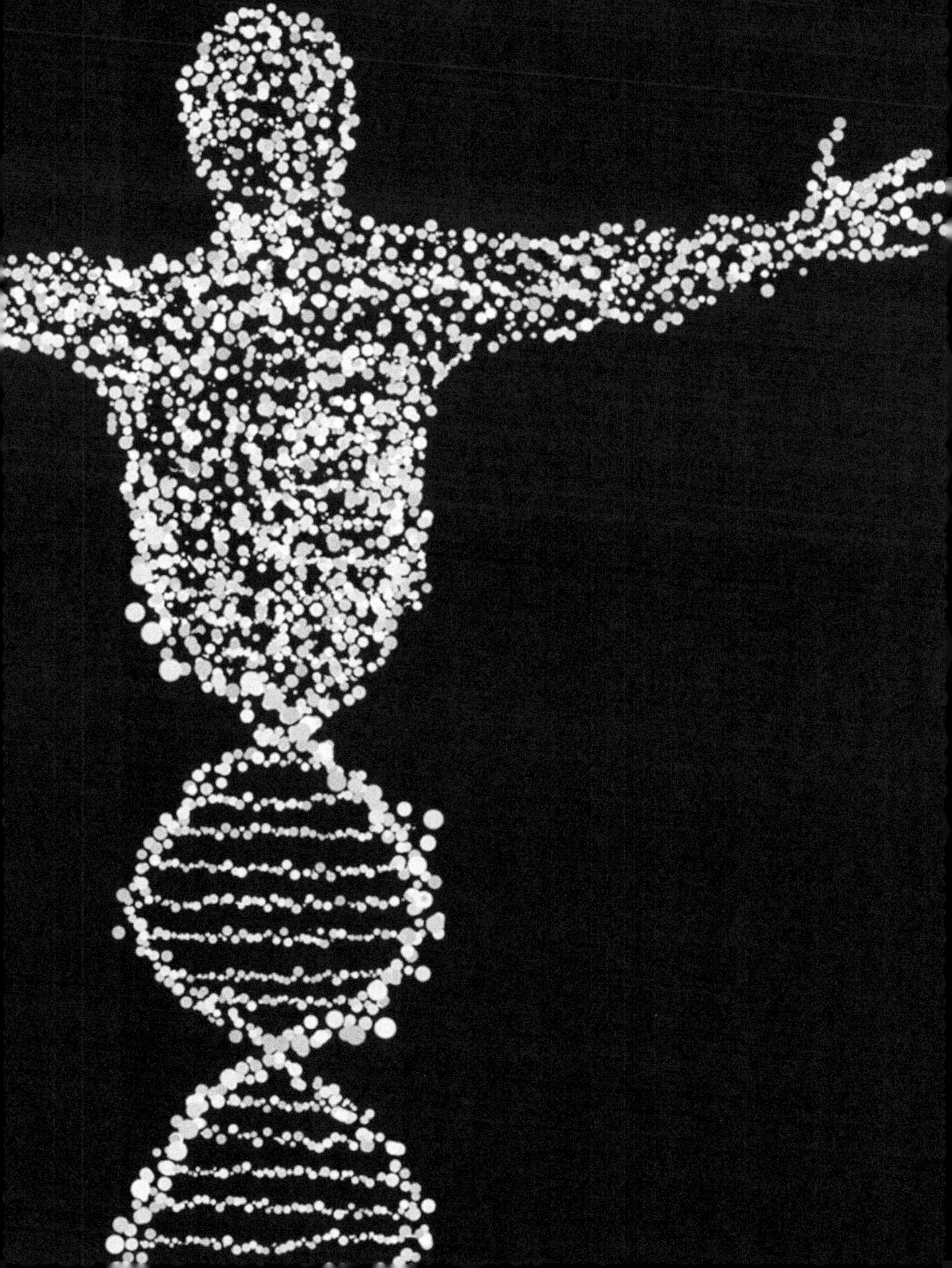

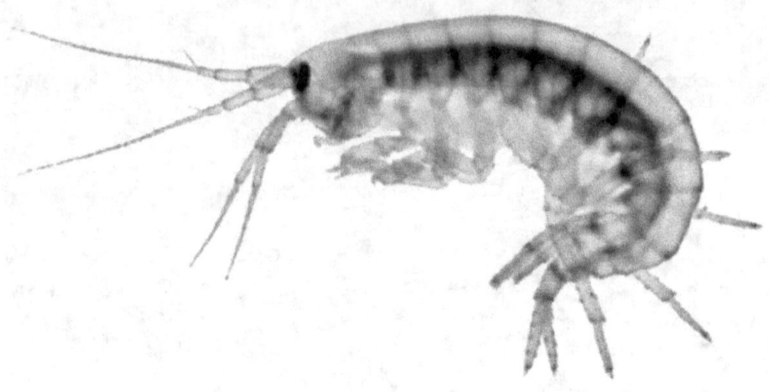

Prescribing for Shrimps

Shrimps kept in sea water laced with the level of fluoxetine currently found in their natural habitat change their behaviour. Dr Alex Ford of Portsmouth University found that instead of seeking cover from predators under rocks, they swim towards light. So human drugs may trigger behaviour changes which could unbalance the ecosystem.

What happens to all the medication we prescribe? It's a challenge to find out.

As we know, a lot isn't ever taken. In one survey, only 18% of people said they completed courses of antibiotics. Unused pharmaceuticals should be returned to a pharmacy. They are then incinerated. In hospital, end of problem. But in the community, probably only 25% of unused prescriptions find their way back to a pharmacist. People usually throw unwanted medication into the household waste or flush it down the toilet.

Either way, it can end up in the environment.

Household waste goes to the dump. Landfill sites in UK have rubber liners, so their contents are contained. But inevitably there are leaks, so chemicals seep into ground water. Once there, they may decompose into who-knows-what-possibly-toxic compounds.

Any drug, whether excreted through the kidneys or the gut or thrown into a British toilet, goes to a sewage treatment works. There, waste water is treated to make it safe to discharge into the environment. These processes also treat water from industry and agriculture, so they have to cope with a huge range of contaminants, some potentially very toxic and in large concentrations. Once treated, the solids (sludge) and the cleaned-up water are discharged onto the land or into rivers or the sea. Any chemicals they still contain may then find their way to the reservoirs and aquifers. That's where most of our drinking water come from; further treatment makes it safe to drink.

Until very recently drugs were the least of the Drinking Water Inspectorate's concerns. DWI was far more worried about particles – no-one wants murk in their glass of water – heavy metals and pathogenic micro-organisms. But twenty years ago someone started asking other questions. And scientists started doing tests.

In clinical practice, levels of anticonvulsants, performance-enhancing drugs and illegal substances are routinely measured, but it's a different matter to test drinking water for tiny quantities of the thousands of drugs we prescribe, let alone their metabolites. Nevertheless the evidence that exists is reassuring. Though many drugs can be detected in treated water, they have never been found at anything near a harmful level.

Research has asked other interesting questions. Can you trace the usage of drugs in a community through their concentrations in waste water? By looking at prescribing data for an area it is possible to estimate the likely consumption of those medications. It is much more difficult to hazard a guess about over-the-counter pharmaceuticals, and almost impossible to calculate usage of illicit drugs. But it has proved possible to estimate communities' usage of some drugs from the concentrations in their sewers. The cocaine levels in waste water from different districts of Barcelona provide useful information about patterns of cocaine consumption in the city.

There are complications. Heavy rains can overwhelm sewage treatment plants and when raw sewage is discharged, drug levels will be higher. The level in our environment of drugs such as antihypertensives is steady throughout the year round. But what about drugs which are used very widely for a brief time? Just as far more thyme and sage appear in American sewers at Thanksgiving, waste water will reflect events. Had the bird flu pandemic turned serious, how much Tamiflu would have reached our water, and what effect might it have had? We don't know. Will micro-organisms exposed to the antibiotics which remain in treated water develop resistance? We don't know. Meanwhile, one way or another, from agriculture, from landfill, from leaky sewers, from treated water, we are dumping an ever more complex soup of pharmacologically active chemicals into our environment.

And we aren't the only living things on the planet. India's

vulture population has plummeted since vets started prescribing diclofenac for cattle. It turns out that cow carcasses contain enough diclofenac for vultures to develop renal failure. It is now well established that 'endocrine disruptors' – which come from many sources besides HRT – can affect the sexual development of amphibians, reptiles and fish. It's not just the anglers who are concerned. And remember those shrimps, putting their lives at risk by swimming towards the light.

Here in Britain our drinking water may be free of other people's Prozac, but the volume of prescriptions goes ever upwards. What can we do about it? The less that goes into the environment the better, which probably means developing water treatment processes specifically designed to remove medications. A campaign to explain to people why they should return unwanted drugs to pharmacies would help. And what happens to shrimps and vultures should matter to us. We aren't just prescribing for Mrs Jones; we are also prescribing for shrimps.

—NASGP August 2012

POSTSCRIPT (January 2015): Since I wrote this article in 2012, further experiments, by Dr Alex Ford and others, have shown that antidepressants in concentrations found in environmental waters can affect molluscs as well as crustaceans and fish. Meanwhile more and more medications are being dispensed.

Photo: The subject of Dr Alex Ford's experiments

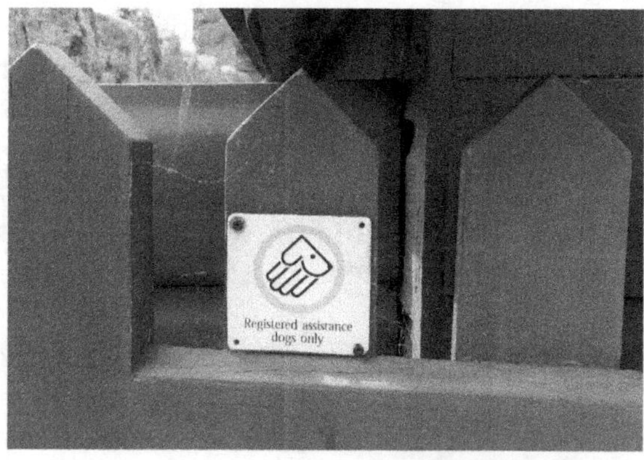

On the Scent of Cancer

Humans are a dog's best friend. Ever since dogs found hunter-gatherers' campsites a good place to scavenge and decided to adopt humans, we have created roles for them: hunting, protecting property, mountain rescue, companionship, and as 'assistance dogs'.

No doubt dogs have been helping people with poor vision for millennia, but it was a German doctor looking after soldiers blinded by gas who in 1916 started the first formal training scheme. Fifteen years later two British dog breeders, Rosamund Bond and Muriel Crooke, trained the first four British guide dogs for the blind. Now there are 5,000.

It isn't a great leap to training dogs to assist people with hearing loss – there are 900 deaf-dog partnerships. Dogs also help people with neurological and degenerative diseases, or seriously disabling injuries – *Hounds for Heroes* provides dogs for ex-servicemen. Dogs can be trained to pick up the TV remote, flush the loo and empty the washing machine. They can retrieve cash from an ATM and help their owner turn over in bed. And they can put their own feeding bowls in the sink and tidy away their own toys. Well ahead of most human teenagers, then.

An assistance dog costs around £50,000 over its working life. Owners have a contract with the charity which supplies their dog, and they contribute what they can to their dogs' care and vets' bills. There is no funding from government. Fortunately the public gives generously to the charities which breed, train and register assistance dogs.

Owner and dog have to be compatible, and not just temperamentally. If you are five feet tall, a poodle would be more your stride than an Alsatian. It's hard work being an assistance dog and they retire early, after about six years, though some stay with their owners as pets.

The owners are in control of their dogs and are responsible for their good behaviour, but a dog needs 'intelligent disobedience': if its owner instructs it to lead him down what he thinks is a flight of steps, his dog has to recognise that it is a precipice and refuse to go on.

Under the 2010 Equality Act registered assistance dogs must be admitted to pubs, cafes and restaurants. Taxi drivers are required to carry guide dogs. Occasionally drivers have tried to refuse, sometimes citing religious prohibitions, though in 2003 the Sharia Council ruled that working dogs are exempt from the proscription on unclean animals.

Airlines too are obliged to provide registered assistance dogs with floor space, normally at no extra charge. In the USA some passengers try to wangle a free place for their pet by waving a doctor's letter, but airlines require to see a dog's registration document, so passengers claiming that their pet pooch is an 'emotional assistance dog' will find themselves paying for Fido to travel in a crate in the hold.

By the way, if you come across someone out with a guide dog, resist the temptation to stroke it – it's at work.

You probably wouldn't be tempted to stroke a sniffer dog, particularly one accompanied by a US marshall. But dogs' olfactory abilities are also put to medical uses. People with a history of anaphylactic reactions can have a dog trained to detect nuts, or a dog can warn its owner of an oncoming hypo or an Addisonian crisis or a life-threatening cardiac arrhythmia. Sufferers and their families can relax their vigilance and live a more normal life. It's a shame for people with epilepsy that there is only weak evidence that dogs can be trained to warn of impending seizures.

Researchers are on the scent of more roles for medical detection dogs. A study in the BMJ in 2012 showed that a trained beagle identified *Clostridium difficile* in stool samples with 100% sensitivity and specificity, and its results were nearly as good when it was taken on the ward to sniff patients. An unorthodox way of overcoming the current delays in diagnosis?

There are many anecdotes of dogs suddenly and repeatedly pawing or nosing their owner's breast, worrying her to the point that she goes to see her GP and a breast cancer is discovered. Research is now providing evidence that dogs can detect signs of malignancy, at least *in vitro*. In 2004 the BMJ published a trial which showed that dogs sniffing urine samples did better than chance at identifying the patient with bladder cancer.

What are dogs detecting? It is known that some cancers produce unusual volatile compounds. How specific are these molecules and can they be identified and used for screening? Milton Keynes Hospital and the charity *Medical Detection Dogs* have permission for a trial of dogs' ability to detect urological cancers from the urine of 3,000 people. If the results are as good as the pilot trials, dogs will be a lot better at screening than PSA tests.

However accurate they prove to be, the NHS is not going to be putting dogs on the pathology department payroll. It just isn't practical. But the hope is that if dogs are detecting cancer-specific compounds, scientists can identify them and develop an electronic nose. So dogs are leading us along the way to earlier and more efficient detection, and perhaps from there to insights into the biology of cancer and to new and more effective treatments.

—NASGP August 2016

POSTSCRIPT (December 2017): Now assistance rats are starting to reduce the four million cases of undetected TB and so prevent avoidable deaths. People infected with TB give off an odour. It is hard for humans to detect but in Tanzania pouched rats are being trained to identify the smell in heat-treated sputum samples. The samples are transferred by motorbike from clinics to labs supported by APOPO, a Belgian NGO, where in 20 minutes a 'HeroRAT' can check 100 samples, a job that takes a human four days. Conventional microscopy has a detection rate of 20% but rats miss very few cases. Positive tests are validated and clinics receive the results within 24 hours. So treatment can be started promptly. APOPO is also supporting training rats to detect land mines.

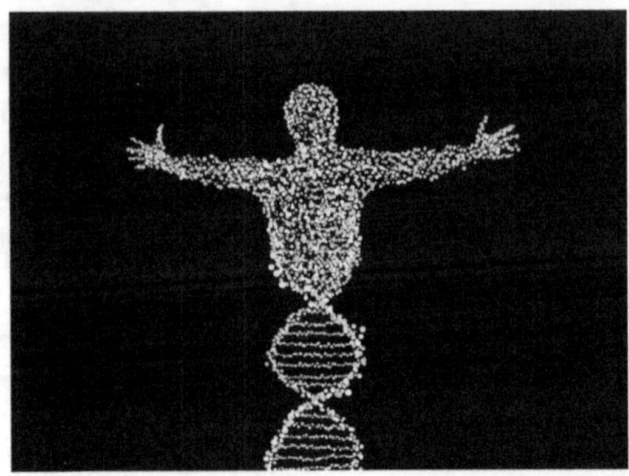

Why Get Your Genome Sequenced?

I confess I don't fully understand what sequencing the human genome means for us. Somewhere between the Secret Of Life and a tall story, it appears. Molecular biology, which for 20 years has been on the A level syllabus, wasn't discovered when I was in the sixth form. It was so simple then: there was Mendel and there were Crick and Watson, and they more or less explained everything.

Now we have mitochondrial DNA, not then known to school text books. We have junk DNA, more respectfully known as non-coding DNA now it is widely thought to have functions we don't yet understand. Since it comprises 98% of our genome, that's a huge potential influence. Then there is epigenetics, which explains – in part – why identical twins reared together don't always have the same illnesses, careers and taste in boy friends. Add the enormous effect of environment and lifestyle, and for most of us most of the time what determines our lives has more to do with our phenotype and our environment than our genotype.

Members of the public are already having key genetic markers in their genome sequenced. Advertisements invite them to investigate their ancestry. Y chromosomes being very stable, men, for as little as $199 for 20 markers, can identify hitherto unknown relatives around the world, sharing information through a database. Or they may discover that someone they thought a blood relative isn't, so this interesting hobby is not without a potential to harm. You can have a test to find out if you have genes from exotic races, but until more genomes have been sequenced you won't know whether you are glamorously unusual in having, say, Neanderthal genes or whether everyone else round the dinner party table has them too.

The most common clinical reason for finding out your genetic status is on behalf of someone else, someone as yet unborn or not yet conceived. Counselling and testing in communities at high risk of genetic disease has greatly reduced the incidence of Tay Sachs disease in Ashkenazi Jewish communities and thalassaemia in Cyprus. In India, parents are urged to match thalassaemia tests rather than horoscopes when considering their children's marriage partners. But 'blue sky' testing of everyone for a wide range of genetic conditions would be costly and, as with any screening of low-risk populations, likely to create anxiety rather than avoid disease.

Genome sequencing will change cancer screening and treatment. Till now it has not been possible to predict whether men with prostate cancer will die with it or of it. Now we know that 16 single-nucleotide polymorphisms (SNPs) are associated with aggressive disease, so in future it will be easier to determine who needs aggressive treatment. And their SNPs will help to determine which 20% of the women with a BRCA gene don't develop breast cancer. Angelina Jolie may have reduced her risk by 95%, but major surgery is not without dangers, so determining these SNPs will provide valuable guidance.

Targeted cancer treatments – drugs designed for specific cancer abnormalities – may not be the magic bullet they first appeared to be, but as cancer genetics develops they are going to make a huge difference to the survival and quality of life of – let's hope – many cancer patients.

There is some enthusiasm for identifying the alleles which influence warfarin metabolism so that warfarin dosage can be better tailored. Great claims are made for strokes and bleeds prevented. But if warfarin dosage is managed following well-established algorithms, the risk is in any case low. And by the time it is feasible to test all patients, warfarin will be last century's drug.

Testing for specific gene sequences in particular clinical situations clearly has huge potential for good. Mass screening for a group of recessive conditions needs careful consideration of the benefits and costs, both to individuals and to the NHS. Whole genome sequencing is now available with those for a few thousand pounds to spend, and the price will drop. It's good to know, people say, and doctors shouldn't stand in the way of patients knowing about themselves. But commercial companies have an interest in people investing in gene sequencing. Some offer pre-test counselling, but many are quiet about the downsides and have no wish to pick up the pieces. The real cost is much more than the price of the test, and what you get is not knowledge but information.

A full genome sequence is like a very thick Russian novel with long chapters on obscure aspects of Russian history. And it's in Russian. And I can't help you interpret it since I don't speak Russian. Even the genome scientists only know a few phrases.

We GPs already struggle to help patients manage the anxiety of not-quite-normal screening tests, and we worry about advising patients with slightly raised risks of ischaemic heart disease. When genome sequencing takes off there will be a lot of fretting. Genetic counselling is a specialised task and not something we are currently trained to do. And it takes a lot of time. Many people understand – more or less – single gene problems like haemophilia, but most conditions are influenced by multiple alleles and SNPs. Judging the clinical significance of these is still in its infancy. And, outside the betting shop, understanding risk is, as we know, very poor.

Gene sequencing provides huge opportunities for prevention and management of disease. And commerce is going to have a huge interest in our genes, to target sales, to weight our insurance, to decide whether we are too risky to employ. We have some time to absorb the implications and to work out how we live with them. Meanwhile, a family tree tells most of us a lot about how our genetic inheritance may influence our lives, and we GPs should bear in mind that, whatever their genetic inheritance, the best thing anyone can do for their health is to stop smoking.

—*NASGP August 2013*

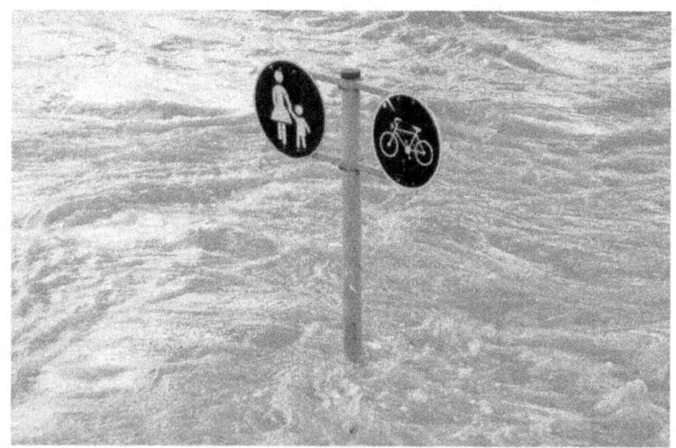

Climate Change Can
Seriously Damage Your Health

Almost a third of those who responded to a recent BMJ poll thought that climate change is not a matter for doctors. Had the doubters been at the Royal College of Physicians' conference on climate change in January, they could not have escaped the impact it will have on health.

Global warming is creating an unstable, chaotic climate, so its effects are hard to predict. How much human conflict will it generate as the world's billions fight for food and water and flee uninhabitable lands? How will nations respond to the threats to their security? Can nations work together using existing knowledge and technology to avoid the destruction of our civilisation?

In the short term, we in the West can buy our way out of trouble. But others can't. Few Africans have a skiing holiday to forgo. They are already on the margin, and they know it. Even in the poorest countries, people turn on the television and compare their lifestyle with ours. Wealthier nations are already feeling the pressure of their discontent. In the USA vigilante groups supplement the border patrols along the Rio Grande. Australia is strengthening its marine defence against southeast Asian immigration. Spain, too, is investing in more powerful maritime patrol vessels, the better to pick up rafts overloaded with Africans hoping to make it to the Canaries and a better life. India is building a 4,500 km wall (two-thirds of the length of the Great Wall of China) to keep out the Bangladeshis fleeing their submerging country. Access to resources already contributes to the drift to cities and to armed conflicts like Dafur and the Middle East, and it will get much, much worse as billions of people try to crowd into the diminishing habitable areas of the globe.

It is not just humans who will be displaced. Already, tick-borne diseases are found at latitudes and altitudes where they never occurred before. Southern Europe's 50-year freedom from malaria is likely to end. And in a world increasingly crowded and lacking adequate water supplies, diarrhoeal disease will be rampant.

How do we tackle a planet-wide threat? We have no history of international co-operation on the scale required. In Hollywood, the world's nations forget their differences when the spaceships arrive. But we are living in an environmental disaster of our own making. We squabble while Amazonia burns, hoping, perhaps, that technology yet again can save us from ourselves. But it will be 20 years before all the damage done by today's level of greenhouse gases is manifest and every year the scale of the problem escalates.

China is rapidly becoming the world's leading source of CO_2, and that is before most of its burgeoning middle class switch from bicycles to cars, take foreign holidays, bathe more than once a week and start using disposable nappies. After a generation of starvation, many Chinese families can now enjoy dining out. But increasing meat consumption is another stress on China's environment, already struggling to provide enough fuel and water. However, it is salutary to remember that a significant portion of China's CO_2 is incurred making cheap consumer goods for the West. If you add the contribution represented by Chinese-made imports, Britain's carbon footprint increases fourfold, and to judge by the number of Primark carrier bags in Oxford Street the British public is not yet ready to sacrifice a cheap T-shirt to save the environment.

As a species, and given time, *Homo sapiens* is very adaptable. But as individuals, most humans cope poorly with sudden disruption. People who live round the Mediterranean are used to 40° summers, but 35,000 northern Europeans died during the 2003 heat wave. Experts predict that within a few decades 40° will be normal summer temperature in London. As the climate becomes more and more unstable, Britain is just one of many countries experiencing devastating floods, Australia's droughts are lasting longer than ever before, the names of Caribbean hurricanes are now extending down the alphabet to W and beyond. Anomalous climatic events are becoming routine, and Hurricane Katrina was a depressing demonstration of how quickly social behaviour and institutions collapse under stress.

We can make our own choices: a 'lodge' sounds less invasive

than a 'hotel' – something which sits lightly on the ground without despoiling it. But how many eco-lodges does it take to create an eco-catastrophe? Everything down to the cocktail shaker may run on solar power, but the aeroplanes which bring the visitors it attracts certainly don't.

Using biofuels may give American motorists a virtuous glow, but the fuel is made from imported maize or soya. So in Mexico people are going hungry because they can no longer afford to make tortillas, and Brazilian forests which buffer CO_2 are being destroyed to plant soya.

Exchanging your Chelsea tractor for a Smart, or even for the most energy-efficient 4-wheel-drive, will help your exchequer and the world's, as will following former Minister of Health Edwina Currie's advice to put on a sweater rather than turning up the thermostat. But it seems rather small beer. We are told that turning off standby lights will power hospitals, but it's a chore and doesn't dramatically reduce our fuel bills. And is it worth it when you look out of the window and see office blocks ablaze with lights 24 hours a day?

Perhaps this is one area where doctors can help. We are still opinion leaders. Let's see fewer staff cars in the surgery car park, more press features about surgery buildings designed with environmental economy in mind, more talk about the medical effects of climate change. Even the increase in allergy as the growing season lengthens may make news. We can then move on to the problems that pestilence and conflict and psychological breakdown will bring if we don't think fast and constructively and together about them. We can press governments to set a visible lead and to introduce policies which will lever businesses and organisations like the NHS and individuals towards carbon-neutral behaviour.

Next time you ring to say "I'm stuck in traffic", remember that you *are* the traffic. Fewer vehicles on the roads would not only reduce CO_2, but also decrease noise, pollution, respiratory disease and trauma. It would promote exercise. Perhaps children would again be able to play safely in the roads. And it would improve the environment. When I go for a walk round the block, I don't choose the road where all the front gardens have been converted to hard standing for cars. I turn left so I can enjoy the camellias and the daffodils behind the garden gates. Preserving beauty is not the least of the benefits of caring for our environment.

—NASGP April 2008

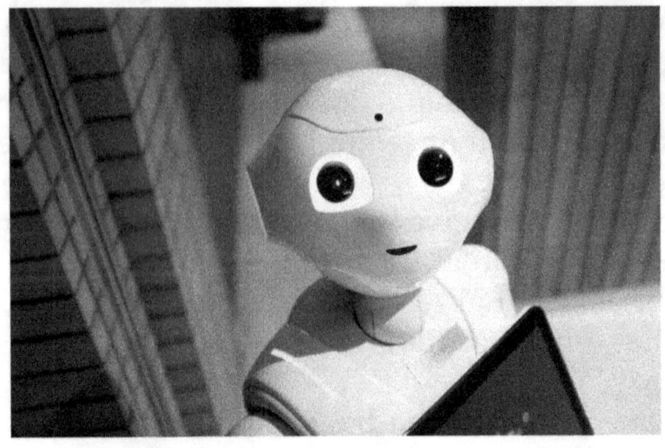

I, Robot BM BCh (Oxon)

How long before machines are cleverer than we are? The first robots were clockwork novelties. Now robots – named for the Russian word *robotnic*, meaning worker – can outperform humans at ever more tasks.

But robots are specialists. They don't have our versatility – yet. They can't yet do what every child can do – transfer learning to a new context. A human trumpeter could make a fist of playing a clarinet, but a robot would have to be reprogrammed. It might be a world-beater at Go but it couldn't play Snap.

Making robots which can perform as well as humans, whether it be at walking, seeing, or thinking, involves understanding how humans walk, see and think. Nature is hard to emulate. But, remember those lumbering movie robots? They've upped their game. Now that we understand the complex mechanics of human ambulation it is possible to build robots which walk like we do, even over rough surfaces.

Robots' 'eyes' can follow humans and even mimic their expressions, but they don't yet see the way we do. When engineers have cracked the saccadic movements of human vision, maybe a housekeeper robot will be able to tell whether that white stuff on the carpet is cocaine or marshmallow and so be able to clean it up without making a worse mess.

Google's DeepMind has analysed the neural basis of transferring learning and has recently overcome, at least partially, the robots' problem of 'catastrophic forgetting'. So future robots will be cleverer. (It is perhaps comforting to know that as they become more human in their capabilities their joints wear out and their backs give them problems.)

Clever robots are now supporting human health professionals, though not yet supplanting them. Robots can perform complex surgical procedures, but only under the control of a human surgeon. They can read mammograms quickly and reliably, but they can't break bad news to patients. Toyota's human support robots can pick up a dropped phone and give it to a bedridden client, but can they give a friendly word and ask about the patient's cat?

Well, they're getting there. 'Social robots' can sometimes succeed where humans fail. Zora is the size of a small person. Institutionalised elderly people take her under their wing and respond better to her encouragement to join activities than the entreaties of a human organiser. Child-sized Zeno has humanoid features. Children with autism find him fascinating and less threatening than coping with human emotions; by interacting with Zeno they can gradually become more comfortable with human social interaction.

But we still don't really understand consciousness and emotional intelligence – the things that make us human. If we don't understand our own consciousness, how can we build a conscious robot?

Will this gulf be bridged by cybernetic organisms – humans who have integrated technology into their bodies? Despite dictionaries' definitions, cyborgs are not creatures of science fiction. We have always modified ourselves: tattoos and piercing for adornment or ritual, compensating for deficiencies with spectacles or joint replacements or pacemakers. Neil Harbisson was born with achromatopsia (no colour vision), but now 'hears' colours via an electronic antenna implanted in his skull. So he's a cyborg, and as long ago as 2004 he persuaded the UK Passport Office that the device was part of him, so should feature in his passport photograph. How different is this from a cochlea implant? And even a conventional hearing aid can become an extension of its user's brain – they function as one unit.

Citizen hackers are taking medical developments into their own hands. Several hundred diabetics have found security loopholes in their continuous glucose monitors and insulin pumps. They have inserted their own predictive algorithms to achieve much more physiological control of their diabetes. The industry is now catching up, working on the commercial development of an artificial pancreas.

Modifications to address health problems can be controversial –

gene therapy for mitochondrial disease for example, or deep brain stimulation treatment for Parkinson's or Tourette's or locked-in syndrome – yet some cyborgs are taking body modification even further. Natural selection generates good-enough solutions to problems, they point out, but why settle for good-enough when we can now improve on nature?

If your colour sense depends not on your retinal cells, but on an electronic device, why not do as Neil Harbisson has and set it to 'see' infrared and ultraviolet? Or hack your hearing aid so you can hear Wi-Fi? Or implant devices which give a buzz when you face north, or when there is an earth tremor, or when the wind is in the east?

Our physical and digital identities are already merging, and cyborgs see themselves as the vanguard of the post–human age, when we change ourselves rather than our environment. Why pollute the planet with light if we can improve our night vision? Why risk losing a smart card when you could implant its chip so you pay for your bus journey or your coffee or sign on to the NHS net by waving your hand over the reader? Why stop with electronics? Why not try to improve your intellectual capacity by hacking your gut microbiome?

There will be problems. Humans are so successful because they are versatile. Making yourself exceptional will have trade-offs: blades may enable you to qualify for an Olympic sprint but they aren't a patch on a multipurpose prosthesis for doing a spot of gardening.

And who's responsible if citizen hacking goes wrong? If you can tamper with your own device, who else can hack it and take control of your health or your motivation or your affect? Could cyborgs use their transhuman capacities to dominate the rest of us?

We want robots working for us, not us for them. Robots will certainly take on more health care roles, but until they can read suppressed emotions, general practitioners are sure of a job. Meanwhile medical developments and personal experimentation will turn more of us into cyborgs. Look out for surprises.

—*NASGP May 2017*